Children with Cochlear Implants in Educational Settings

School-Age Children Series

Series Editor
Nickola Wolf Nelson, Ph.D.

Children of Prenatal Substance Abuse
Shirley N. Sparks, M.S.

What We Call Smart: Literacy and Intelligence
Lynda Miller, Ph.D.

Whole Language Intervention for School-Age Children
Janet Norris, Ph.D., and Paul Hoffman, Ph.D.

School Discourse Problems, Second Edition
Danielle Newberry Ripich, Ph.D., and
Nancy A. Creaghead, Ph.D.

Supporting Language Learning in Everyday Life
Judith Felson Duchan, Ph.D.

Including Students with Severe Disabilities in Schools
Stephen N. Calculator, Ph.D., and
Cheryl M. Jorgensen, Ph.D.

Children with Cochlear Implants in Educational
Settings
Mary Ellen Nevins, Ed.D., and Patricia M. Chute, Ed.D.

Children with Cochlear Implants in Educational Settings

Mary Ellen Nevins, Ed.D.
Kean College of New Jersey
Union, New Jersey

Patricia M. Chute, Ed.D.
Cochlear Implant Center
Manhattan Eye, Ear & Throat Hospital
New York, New York

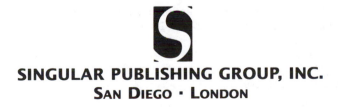

SINGULAR PUBLISHING GROUP, INC.
SAN DIEGO · LONDON

Singular Publishing Group, Inc.
4284 41st Street
San Diego, California 92105-1197

19 Compton Terrace
London, N1 2UN, UK

© 1996 by Singular Publishing Group, Inc.

Typeset in 10/12 Palatino by So Cal Graphics
Printed in the United States of America by BookCrafters

Library of Congress Cataloging-in-Publication Data

Nevins, Mary Ellen
    Children with cochlear implants in educational settings / Mary Ellen Nevins, Patricia M. Chute.
      p. cm.—(School-age children series)
    Includes bibliographical references and index.
    ISBN 1-56593-160-2
    1. Cochlear implants. 2. Hearing impaired children—Education.
3. Hearing impaired children—Rehabilitation. I. Chute, Patricia
M. II. Title. III. Series.
    [DNLM: 1. Cochlear Implant—in infancy & childhood. 2. Child,
Exceptional—education. WV 274 N528c 1995]
RF305.N48   1995
618.92'097882—dc20
DNLM/DLC
for Library of Congress   95-36998
                                                   CIP

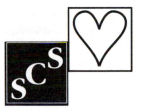

Contents

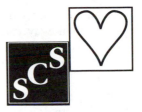

Foreword

I love this book. "Sure," you say, "not a surprising comment from a Series Editor." Well, let me count the reasons why this book by Mary Ellen Nevins and Patricia M. Chute not only makes a perfect fit to the School-Age Children Series, but a significant contribution to the needs of children with cochlear implants.

Consistent with the goals of the series, *Children with Cochlear Implants in Educational Settings* is designed to educate readers about a particular area of concern and to engage them in problem solving to reduce future need for concern. This particular book is grounded in a context that recognizes both the concerns of the Deaf community about cochlear implants as a treatment for deafness and the ongoing story of development of the technology. The material is up-to-date without being dated—not an easy feat for a work tied closely to technological advances.

Even with its clear explanations of socio-political, technological, and theoretical underpinnings, the book is applied in focus, full of suggestions that will stimulate specific ideas about "what to do on Monday morning" (the classic test of practicality). The blending of theory and application is accomplished by providing liberal examples, including sample instructional dialogues, and by anticipating questions that parents and teachers ask, as well as providing specific intervention ideas and strategies.

Nevins and Chute's book also exemplifies several themes that thread their way throughout the series. First, it is consistent with a view of collaboration as a desired mode of problem solving.

This emphasis appears particularly in the authors' focus on the role of educational consultants who build collaborative connections among parents; educational teams in the settings where children are served every day; and medical teams where cochlear implants are considered, surgically placed if appropriate, and tuned and monitored. Second, this book is consistent with a view of children as individuals whose needs are shaped by multiple contexts that change over time. Nevins and Chute do this by considering children's diverse home cultures as well as special classrooms and mainstream school cultures. They are particularly good at offering suggestions for curriculum-based intervention activities that promise to be highly relevant for meeting children's needs, whether at preschool age or in the upper elementary or secondary years. A third unifying theme, which appears both in this book and in the series, is change—change in the way children with cochlear implants use auditory input for making sense and learning, and change in the home and educational contexts that will support them in getting maximal assistance from the technology. The final unifying theme of both the book and the series is relevance. All of the books in this series are aimed at helping professionals become more relevant to meeting the real-life needs of children. This book is an outstanding example of a clinical philosophy that emphasizes the importance of using content and contexts for assessment and intervention that are relevant to the needs of children, particularly in classroom settings.

Perhaps the strongest element of the text is its ability to convey a philosophy and set of strategies for facilitating auditory development among children with cochlear implants. As the authors clearly communicate, no longer is it enough to hold a view of auditory *training*, in which children were taught *to* listen; today's view, and the message of this book, is one of auditory *learning*, in which children are shown how to learn *through* listening. That is a message that promises to make a difference for children with cochlear implant and their families.

Nickola Wolf Nelson, Ph.D.
Series Editor

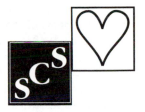

Preface

The cochlear implant is a recognized technology which provides deaf children with access to auditory signals previously inaccessible through traditional amplification. Although initial outcome measures focused on the auditory perceptual changes of children who received implants, the secondary goals realized from implantation manifested themselves in the classroom environment. Here, the application of new listening skills appeared to make a substantial difference in learning style. The important role that the educational setting plays in maximizing benefit from the implant has yet to be addressed. The goal of this book is to provide a reader-friendly introduction to working with children with cochlear implants in their school settings. We have attempted to fill a need recognized out of our many years experience in working with parents and school-based personnel. This book is written for the practicing school professional, hospital and clinical personnel, professionals in training, and parents interested in the educational aspects of implantation. It provides a review of the knowledge and skills needed to help a child maximize the potential of the cochlear implant.

In writing this book, we have made a conscious departure from other books on cochlear implants by exploring the issues that are seldom addressed elsewhere. Events, such as the choice of a cochlear implant, occur in a context. Each and every family's individual circumstances which lead them to choose implantation as an option for their child cannot be known. However, some generalizations can be made about the larger social, political, and educational contexts in which the decision to implant takes place. Chapter 1 addresses the implications of the social and political issues surrounding implantation. An educational orientation to cochlear implants is continued in Chapter 2. Here, a child-centered approach to the cochlear implant process is explored. The implant is introduced as a medical procedure with important educational ramifications. This creates a need for articulation between hospitals and schools, two institutions that have little history in forming cooperative relationships. The utility of an educational consultant model to help bridge the gap from hospital to school is presented. In Chapter 3, a description of how the cochlear implant functions, details regarding the surgical procedure, and photographs illustrating the particular features of the available devices are presented. Once a working knowledge of the device has been established, the guidelines for candidacy selection are outlined in Chapter 4. This is perhaps the most important chapter in the book, for it is our belief that a properly selected candidate is the foundation on which performance expectations for the device can best be met. The role of the school and school professionals in helping a center evaluate candidacy is highlighted. The Children's Implant Profile developed by the staff of the Cochlear Implant Center of Manhattan Eye, Ear & Throat Hospital is detailed in this chapter. In Chapter 5, attention is focused on the changing needs of the parents during the three phases of implantation: the evaluation phase, the surgical phase, and the rehabilitative phase. The various support activities necessary during these three phases are outlined as well.

The realities of designing a management program for a child with an implant are identified in Chapter 6. This chapter provides a blueprint for the development of a postimplant program for the child returning to his home school. Steps for performing daily equipment checks and trouble-shooting the device are presented in this chapter as well. In Chapter 7 the important auditory work that follows implant surgery is described. Basic terms such as *detection* and *discrimination* are reviewed, as is the more advanced concept of auditory comprehension. Eight premises which serve as the foundation for any auditory learning program are presented.

Chapters 8, 9, and 10 address the needs of the young implant recipient, the school-age recipient, and the teenage user, respectively. Overall management and rehabilitation strategies specific to these three age groups are presented. A unit-based habilitation protocol is recommended for the preschool and elementary-age child; it is outlined using actual classroom material to serve as an example of how to adapt the protocol to a teacher's particular curriculum. Recommendations for motivating teenagers for the necessary postimplant rehabilitation are offered in Chapter 10.

Performance data on the use of the implant are presented in Chapter 11 in a practical manner so that information is clear and understandable. Also of interest in this chapter is the delineation of a broad time line for the achievement of auditory skills. This knowledge will enable teachers to have appropriate expectations for their students and alert them to irregularities that may signal a need for intervention by the implant center. In Chapter 12, the issue of mainstreaming is addressed, especially as a viable educational alternative for the child successfully using the cochlear implant. Finally, each appendix in this book provides practical information for both teachers and parents. These materials include sample letters, device troubleshooting guides, a checklist to monitor mainstream performance, and a parent dictionary. The glossary defines many of the technical terms which are necessary for the teacher to use and understand. These appendixes and glossary provide a dimension to the book that the teacher and parent will find most helpful when seeking sensible information in the area of cochlear implantation.

Cochlear implantation may open the door to educational choices that parents may not have previously considered making. The final impact that the cochlear implant will have on the field of deaf education represents the underlying theme of this book and is the question which may only be answered with the passage of time.

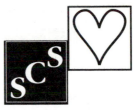

Acknowledgments

We would like to acknowledge the support and input of the many individuals who made this text possible. First and foremost is Dr. Simon C. Parisier whose foresight in recognizing the role of the educator on the cochlear implant team created the environment in which a book such as this could be written. With the financial support of the Children's Hearing Institute, the educational consultant model could be implemented without undue burden to families and schools, thus proving the wisdom of his vision. This model enabled us to meet many school-based professionals, including Dr. Laura McKirdy at the Lake Drive School for Deaf and Hard of Hearing Children. Her confidence in the team at Manhattan Eye, Ear & Throat Hospital prompted an introduction to Nickola Wolf Nelson, the series editor.

Needless to say, the input and cooperation of the many teachers, parents, and children provided the entire educational team the experiences which drove the content of this book. They are to be thanked as well. Finally, we thank Amy L. Popp, whose dedication and attention to detail powered us through the final hours of manuscript preparation.

Dedication

This book is dedicated to our own children
Nell, Bridget, and Colleen O'Leary and
Cara and Robert Chute Jr.

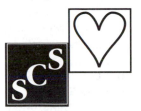

Prologue

Amy Turner was a healthy child, seldom visiting the doctor except for routine well visits. At 13 months, she was walking, able to understand a number of short sentences, and had a few recognizable words in her vocabulary. She was the youngest of three girls in a traditional family setting. Soon after her first birthday, Amy contracted a minor cold with some flu-like symptoms. After a day or two of treatment with acetaminophen, she appeared to be getting better. Suddenly, her fever recurred and her symptoms worsened. Within 24 hours, she was hospitalized with the diagnosis of hemophilus influenza meningitis. Her parents sat at her bedside for 2 days while she was in a coma. Although the Turners were relieved when Amy emerged from her coma, it soon became obvious that something was terribly wrong. No longer would Amy calm to her mother's voice. Nor would she play along when her father attempted to entertain her with a game of peek-a-boo. She did not alert to the hospital sounds around her. When her parents reported this to the pediatrician, she suggested that Amy's hearing be tested as soon as she was well enough to participate in the procedure. In addition to the possibility of a hearing problem, Amy could no longer walk. She could not stand without falling over and could not take a step without assistance. Consequently, she reverted to crawling as a means of getting around. Her few recognizable words were now difficult to understand. It seemed as though the sound of her voice was different too.

Two weeks later, Amy was scheduled for a series of appointments. These included a meeting with an otologist and an audiologist. During those 2 weeks, Amy's parents and sisters noticed her continued lack of responsiveness to any sound. Her attempts to talk sounded more like screeches than words. By the time the Turners met with the audiologist, they were fraught with guilt and anxiety. The test results confirmed their worst fears—Amy was deaf. In those few minutes, the family's world turned upside down. The ramifications of a profound hearing loss were unknown to these parents. The audiologist made some recommendations, but the Turners hardly heard a word. Confused, angry, and distraught, they returned home to adjust to the new information about their daughter. During the course of the next few weeks there was much information to be learned, many decisions to be made and additional appointments to be kept. The Turners tried to read as much as they could about deafness and the educational options available for Amy. Would they choose English or American Sign Language, oral communication or manual communication, the Deaf world or the hearing world for their child?

Slowly, but surely, decisions were made. Amy received physical therapy to help correct her balance problems. Over time, she regained the motor skills she had lost after the meningitis. With regard to her educational needs as a deaf child, Amy's parents chose an early intervention program which employed a total communication philosophy. The entire family enrolled in sign language classes to help Amy learn to communicate at home. Two powerful hearing aids were prescribed for her. She wore them without complaint but her response to sound appeared minimal. Amy learned signs readily and used them to communicate her needs and wants throughout the next year. But the Turners were determined to help their daughter to use speech as well as sign language to communicate.

One evening while watching a program on television about individuals with profound deafness, a new device, known as the cochlear implant, was discussed. Curious about this latest technology, the Turners called the television station and received more information about whom to contact. They also called their pediatrician and audiologist who had only limited information about the device. While there was research information about the implant, the Turners had difficulty understanding the technical literature. They wanted to know how the implant worked and how it would impact their daughter's education. Since the technology was relatively new, many of their questions were unanswerable. Eventually, the Turners located an implant facility which housed a team of experienced professionals who could provide information and support.

The staff at the implant center was able to answer many of the Turner's questions and were sensitive to their needs. They had seen many families of children with profound deafness who were concerned about their child's communication ability. The implant center staff gave the Turners names of other parents whose children had already received the device. Sharing experiences with parents of other children with similar case histories helped the Turners tremendously. Because evaluation for candidacy carried no risks, they began the assessment process. The results indicated that Amy would be a good candidate for a cochlear implant. Armed with the knowledge of the benefits and risks of the implant, and the view of the Deaf community toward it, the Turners chose implantation for their daughter.

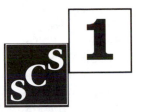

The Social, Political, and Educational Context for Implant Technology

The emergence of new technologies that impact our everyday lives is often greeted by a wary public with caution or skepticism. These might include automated teller machines, the microwave oven, the video cassette recorder, and computer technology with CD-ROMS. Advances in medical technology may meet with the same caution; however, the government requires that they undergo much more rigorous scrutiny before introduction to the public. The process of government regulation has been established for the safety of the general population. It is during this time that the risks and benefits of the technology are examined, and information concerning the technology's use is communicated to the consumer. With every new advance, comes controversy. The cochlear implant has not been immune from this phenomenon. It has garnered both resounding praise and vehement condemnation.

Pioneers in the medical community have hailed the implant as an advancement in the treatment of individuals with profound deafness. Another group has deemed the implantation of young children "deplorable." This group, the adult Deaf Community, rejects the implant, the medical and educational personnel who work on implant teams, and the individuals, both children and adults, who receive it. Professionals who provide services to potential implant candidates and to recipients of the device should be knowledgeable about the Deaf Community's objections to it. To understand these objections, it is necessary to explore the current social, political, and educational climate surrounding deafness and implantation. Despite the fact that these are complex issues, intricately interwoven, they must be addressed independently. However, these forces interact to create the backdrop against which one must consider issues of acceptance of the cochlear implant.

■□ SOCIAL ISSUES

The field of deafness has been rife with controversy throughout the ages. A dichotomous choice always seems to be offered: oral versus manual communication, American Sign Language versus English, schools for the deaf versus mainstreaming. At the root of the current controversy is yet another dichotomy, deficit versus cultural models of deafness. This battle is waged between the medical and the Deaf[1] communities. The medical establishment, as well as the allied professional community of audiologists, views deafness from the perspective of the medical model, referred to by some as the deficit model. The *medical model* suggests that deafness is the absence of hearing, derived from abnormalities in the function of the ear. As such, deafness is a condition to be diagnosed and treated, with devices to be prescribed and a plan of re/habilitation to be implemented This model is contrasted with the cultural model of deafness. The *cultural model* views deafness as a difference, not a deficit. Those who are deaf form the Deaf Community and are viewed as a language and culture minority in which deafness is normal, not pathological. In fact, this cultural view of deafness has caused the Deaf Community to reject the diagnosis of hearing *impairment* and the label of hearing *impaired*. These terms,

---

[1]Following common convention the term "Deaf" is used when referring to the linguistic and cultural subgroup. The term "deaf" is used when referring to the audiologic description of hearing sensitivity.

according to the Deaf Community, have a negative connotation, that is, unable to hear. The terms *deaf* and *deafness* are preferred because these words, in and of themselves, do not linguistically suggest an inability. They simply label a group and its common denominator.

Like other minority groups, there are a number of characteristics that serve to identify members of the Deaf Community. Chief among the identifying characteristics for the Deaf is their unique language, American Sign Language (ASL). This language is distinctly different from oral languages in general, and different grammatically from English, in particular. ASL is not to be confused with signed English systems currently in use in many schools. Unlike English sign systems, ASL signs are "layered and richly configured" (Lane, 1992, p. 16) to communicate meaning. Sign systems used in educational settings provide a word for word representation of a sentence. Members of the Deaf Community believe that sign systems are an attempt by hearing people to improve upon ASL and make it more like English.

With regard to the cochlear implant, the Deaf Community believes that the implant poses a threat to its very existence. Lane (1992) likened the implant to questionable practices of the past:

> Among the biological means aimed at regulating and ultimately eliminating deaf culture, language and community, cochlear implants have historical antecedents, then, in medical experimentation on deaf children and reproductive regulation on deaf adults. (p. 216)

Further, many Deaf activists believe that the existence of the cochlear implant sends the message that deaf people aren't good enough. They interpret the technology as proof that hearing people "want to eradicate deafness and, by implication, wish that they—Deaf people—didn't exist" (Woodcock, 1992, p. 152). If this is the case then, it is indeed no wonder that the Deaf Community published a position paper denouncing the decision of the Food and Drug Administration (FDA) to approve the marketing of an implant device for children (see Figure 1–1). Although the position of the Deaf Community may appear to be extreme, remarks made by insensitive supporters of and divisive objectors to the device serve to fuel the bitter controversy. Woodcock (1992), in an appeal to her fellow members of the Deaf Community, summarized her belief that:

> The cochlear implant does not represent a threat to Deaf Culture. What is a threat is the Deaf Community's overeagerness to reject prospective members just because . . . their parents chose an implant for them . . . The

Cochlear Implants in Children

A Position Paper of the National Association of the Deaf

Background

On June 27, 1990, the Food and Drug Administration (FDA) approved the marketing of the Nucleus 22-channel cochlear prosthesis for surgical implantation in children aged two through seventeen. (Commercial distribution for postlingually-deafened adults was authorized in 1985; investigational trials began in adolescents, age ten to seventeen, the same year and in young children, age two through nine, in November 1986.) This recent FDA approval of marketing childhood implants, recommended by its Ear, Nose and Throat Devices Panel, was based on a submission by the manufacturer, the Cochlear Corporation, which reported on a total of 200 implanted children, ages two through seventeen, who had bilateral, profound sensorineural deafness.

The position of the National Association of the Deaf

The NAD deplores the decision of the Food and Drug Administration which was unsound scientifically, procedurally, and ethically.

Scientific errors

Implantation of cochlear prosthesis in early-deafened children remains highly experimental. There is no evidence of material benefit from the device in this population and no evaluation of the long-term risks. There is no evidence that the speech perception of these children is materially enhanced but there is evidence that many profoundly deaf children would have better, however limited, speech perception with conventional hearing aids than with implants. There is no evidence that early implanted children will do better at acquiring English than they would with noninvasive aids or with no aid whatsoever. There is no evidence that early-implanted children will have greater educational success than is currently experienced by children of similar circumstances who do not undergo this invasive surgical procedure. The FDA Panel has required the device packaging to include the warning that congenitally deaf children may derive no benefit from the device but the evidence points to the same conclusion for children deafened below the age of three and possibly age five or later.

Current programs of research on cochlear implants with children are conducted without regard to the quality of life that the child will experience as a deaf adult implant user. It is presently unknown whether the implant and the profound commitment of parent and child to aural/oral training that is generally required, will delay the family's acceptance of the child's deafness and their acquisition of sign communication. The impact of the implant and the required aural/oral training on the child's social, intellectual and emotional development and mental health, or on the child's integration into the deaf community, have not been assessed. This failure alone to consider the impact of the implant on the child's future quality of life qualifies the implant programs as highly experimental—just what the World Federation of the Deaf deplored when it resolved, "Implant developments are encouraging for persons deafened after some years of hearing [but] experimentation with young deaf children is definitely not encouraged."

Procedural errors

The FDA erred in failing to obtain formal input from organizations of deaf Americans and from deaf leaders and scholars knowledgeable about the acquisition and use of sign communication and English in deaf children, the psychosocial development and education of deaf children, and the social organization and culture of the American Deaf community. The research evidence makes abundantly clear that early-deafened implanted children will rely on sign communication in school and in much of their lives. Many, perhaps most of these children will become or already are members of the American Deaf Community. Otologists, speech and hearing scientists, manufacturers, parents and members of the FDA staff were all consulted formally by the FDA in arriving at its decision. FDA's failure to consult deaf spokespersons represents, if an oversight, gross ignorance concerning growing up deaf in America, or, if willful, an offense against fundamental American values of individual liberties, cultural diversity and consumer rights.

Ethical errors

Experimentation on children is ethically offensive. New and high technology that entails invasive surgery and tissue destruction is used, not for life saving, but for putative life enhancement. Adults, such as these children will become, when given the option of such prostheses, overwhelmingly decline them. The parents who make the decision for the child are often poorly informed about the deaf community, its rich heritage and promising futures, including communication modes available to deaf people and their families. Far more serious is the ethical issue raised through decisions to undertake invasive surgery upon defenseless children, when the long-term physical, emotional and social impacts on children from this irreversible procedure—which will alter the lives of these children—have not been scientifically established.

Recommendations

The National Association of the Deaf advocates the following course of action:

(1) The Food and Drug Administration should withdraw marketing approval and revise the procedures employed for evaluating proposals for authorization of cochlear implants in children.

(2) The National Institute on Deafness and Other Communicative Disorders (NIDCD) should fund research on the present population of implanted children which will allow a comprehensive assessment of risks and benefits for the child that include educational and family circumstances issues, social adjustment, mental health and quality of life issues. In the meantime, the Institute should not fund any additional implanting of early-deafened children. The Institute should require that research programs related to deaf children involve deaf leaders and experts, in order to get any continuing or new funding. Research programs on childhood cochlear prostheses should measure material enhancement of speech reception and production, such as open-set recognition of ordinary conversation in moderately noisy environments, with and without decisions to undertake invasive surgery upon defenseless children, when the long-term physical, emotional and social impacts on children from this procedure have not been scientifically established.

The National Association of the Deaf will work with the FDA, the National Institute on Deafness and Other Communicative Disorders (NIDCD), hospitals and other organizations on appropriate measures against surgically implanting early-deafened children. Parents should also be provided with printed information concerning organizations of deaf persons in their community and other sources of information about the deaf community, its culture, its language and its heritage. ■

Prepared by the NAD Task Force on Cochlear Implants in Children Dr. Harlan Lane, Chair, Dr. Barbara Brauer, Dr. Larry Fleischer, Joyce Groode, Nathie Marbury and Michael Schwartz, Esq. Approved by the NAD Board of Directors, 2/2/91.

Reprinted from NAD Broadcaster, 3/91.

Figure 1–1

The National Association for the Deaf Position Paper on Cochlear Implants in Children. (From NECCI News 1991, reprinted with permission.)

Deaf Culture would be wise to realize that it has a lot to offer without having to oppress or malign other backgrounds or points of view. (p. 155)

■□ THE POLITICAL CONTEXT

In these times of political activism, it is not surprising that the Deaf Community has found a "voice" to speak to issues of concern to their interests. General dissatisfaction with the education of all children with disabilities led parents, educators, and lawmakers to establish new legal guidelines for teaching children with exceptional needs. The original legislation, known as the Education of All Handicapped Children Act was established in 1975. It was reauthorized in 1990 as IDEA—Individuals with Disabilities Education Act. Attention to the needs of persons with disabilities in occupational and recreational areas, as well as educational activities, led to the passage of the Americans with Disabilities Act (ADA) (1990). While large numbers of Deaf individuals do not see themselves as disabled, they have used this legislation to help them gain access to goods and services in a manner similar to their hearing counterparts. Although the above mentioned legislation represents a national trend toward recognizing the needs of all individuals with differences, the Deaf Community experienced a watershed event that served to unite and solidify them as a political entity in their own right. The political climate of the country created a perfect environment for the Deaf Community to make a statement regarding their presence in society. In March of 1988, national attention was drawn to Washington, DC, not because it is the national political center of the United States, but because it is the home of Gallaudet University, the only liberal arts university in the United States for deaf students.

At that time, Gallaudet was searching for a new president. Of the three final candidates for the position, two were deaf and one was hearing. The Gallaudet community was hopeful that one of the deaf applicants would be appointed. The Board of Directors of the college, comprised of a majority of hearing members, selected the hearing applicant as its candidate. Upon the news of the Board's action, deaf students, faculty, staff, and alumni participated in a protest march to confront the Board. The chairman of the Board attempted to explain the choice by suggesting that a deaf president would be incapable of administering the college in situations which would require functioning in the hearing world. These remarks further outraged the crowd. By the start of the next school day, the students had taken control of key campus administrative buildings. Top-level administrators were refused admittance, so the university was officially closed. After an entire week of rallies and other protest activities, the appointed hearing president resigned, and a deaf president was selected. The chairman of the Board also resigned and the Board membership was reconstituted so that the majority of its members were deaf. All students involved in the protest were free from reprisals. Members of Gallaudet University and the entire Deaf Community saw this as a resounding victory in the cause for Deaf power.

This political action galvanized the Deaf Community and made their presence visible to the rest of the country. Now seen as a special interest group, major political figures seeking political office have begun to court Deaf Community support. Key campaign speeches in large metropolitan areas are seldom made without ASL interpreters present. Although there are a number of quality of life issues that concern the Deaf Community in the political domain, of paramount importance to the Deaf Community is the education of deaf children. It is through the educational system that the language and culture of the Deaf are transmitted.

■□ THE EDUCATIONAL CONTEXT

Historically, the education of deaf children has taken place in residential schools for the deaf (Moores, 1987). In these programs, deaf children attended classes by day and were supervised in living situations during after-school and weekend hours. They returned home for the summer holiday, only to be sent back to the residential school in September. Important social relationships were established in the residential school, and often a large community of adult deaf individuals would cluster in the towns where these schools were located. The country's demographics with regard to deafness contributed to the development of strategically located state schools for the deaf in virtually every state. Broad expansion of state facilities was undertaken in the early 1970s as the children of the rubella epidemic of the late 1960s were identified and enrolled in school programs. Thus, state residential schools for the deaf were a center for education and socialization and a place where enculturation into the Deaf Community could take place. It was in the residential programs that deaf children learned ASL and the values of the Deaf Community.

In addition to the state residential schools, some major metropolitan cities also established schools for the deaf. Because there was a critical mass of deaf children already living in these urban areas, the city schools were more likely to be day programs. Although the combination of residential and day school services was adequate for quite some time, legislation of the mid 1970s, PL 94-142, the Education of All Handicapped Children Act, identified the right of all children with special needs to be educated in the "least restrictive environment." This is interpreted by many as synonymous with mainstreaming, or the education of children with disabilities alongside their nondisabled peers in their local school. As local school districts complied with PL 94-142, small regional and day class programs began cropping up, and a gradual shift in the placement of deaf students could be seen (see Table 1–1). More students were being educated in local programs than in state residential schools. As this trend continues into the 1990s, many state schools are now closing or enrolling students with multiple handicaps. Alumni of these deaf schools are protesting the disappearance of the deaf school experience as they knew it. They argue that deaf children have a right to be educated with their deaf peers in the least restrictive *communicative* environment. Among the items on the political agenda of the Deaf Community is to preserve the state residential school as an educational and cultural center for deaf children.

Of equal if not greater importance to the discussion of where deaf children are to be educated is the question of how they are to be educated. The field of education of deaf children has been indicted for its failure to live up to its expectation and investment. As a group, deaf children continue to lag behind their hearing agemates in reading and academic achievement (Allen, 1986). Although the cause of the lag is another debated topic, a group of linguists from Gallaudet University has suggested that it is due to deaf children's lack of "natural language

TABLE 1–1

Comparison of Enrollments in Schools and Classes for the Deaf in the United States in the Past 20 Years.

	1974[1]	1993–1994[2]
Residential (public and private)	20,564	9,561
Day school for deaf (public and private)	8,073	3,549
Day class	534	30,534

Sources: [1]Adapted from W. Craig and H. Craig (Eds.). (1975). Directory of services for the Deaf, *American Annals of the Deaf, 120*, p. 118. [2]From Center for Assessment and Demographic Studies (1994). Annual survey of deaf and hard of hearing children and youth, 1993–1994. Washington, DC: Gallaudet University.

competence and for communicative access to curricular material" (Johnson, Liddell, & Erting, 1989, p. 1). The natural language in this instance is ASL. Some state residential programs and a number of day programs are experimenting with, or have adopted the use of, ASL as the language of instruction. However, the majority of educational programs are designed to deliver instruction using the English language, regardless of whether that instruction is accomplished in an oral or simultaneous (oral and manual) code.

The language of instruction becomes an issue when evaluating the potential effectiveness of an implant in such a communicative environment. By its very nature, the structure of ASL precludes the simultaneous use of voice. The value of an implant in a silent communicative setting is highly questionable. Although there is a move toward the adoption of ASL in a growing number of programs and schools for the deaf, there is a countermovement toward inclusion of deaf students in classes with their hearing agemates.

Inclusive education, a newly coined term, is a product of the broader special education field. It removes the child from the segregated special class and places him in the regular classroom. It is here that the services of the special education teacher are delivered—either directly or indirectly to the child through consultation to the regular classroom teacher. This contrasts with *mainstreaming* which has historically been defined as placement in the regular classroom without a special education classification.

A number of factors contribute to the feasibility of inclusive education for deaf children; cochlear implant technology may support this trend. With the enhanced listening and speech skills made possible by the implant, deaf children may exhibit the numerous abilities needed for successful regular school placement. Assessing the functioning of children with cochlear implants in regular classrooms requires longitudinal study. Given the recency of cochlear implant technology, many studies of this nature are at their infancy stage.

Longitudinal studies of children with cochlear implants in mainstream placements should address their educational achievements as well as explore their social and emotional well-being. Assessment of educational progress should include the standard measures of reading and mathematics in addition to the development of critical thinking skills. Determining social emotional status can be accomplished either through direct observation or through the use of interviews and/or questionnaires. Because previous studies have found that the social adjustment of deaf children in regular classrooms may be compromised (Antia, 1982; Mertens, 1989), this aspect of mainstream placement for deaf children with implants requires careful attention. Whether regular education placement is labelled inclusive or mainstream, children with implants in these settings need monitoring to ensure success there. In addition, careful study of these children is necessary to add to the body of knowledge regarding the impact of this device on social and academic achievement. In this way, the social, political, and educational context of implantation of children will be driven by data rather than emotion.

■❑ SUMMARY

The cochlear implant is an emerging technology which, like many new technologies, brings with it controversy and resistance. The implantation of deaf children, in particular, must be viewed within the social, political, and educational contexts of deafness and the Deaf Community. Parents must be aware of the controversy surrounding the implant and understand the issues as they relate to individuals who are deaf. Choosing implantation for a young deaf child without the full knowledge of the implications of that choice is ill-advised. Parents, educators, and professionals in the allied fields of audiology and speech-language pathology have a responsibility to educate themselves about the implantation process. Studies which provide data on the social and educational outcomes of children with implants will contribute objective information to the debate of the use of this technology with children.

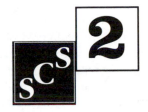

A Child-Centered Approach to the Cochlear Implant Process

The Food and Drug Administration (FDA) is the federal agency responsible for overseeing the introduction of new products into the marketplace. When products are intended for use in both children and adults, the FDA requires a period of product testing in the adult population before allowing its use within the children's market. Such was the case with the cochlear implant. Before the device could be implanted in children, data were gathered on deaf adults to determine the effectiveness of the device. Although many of the findings during the test trials in the adult population were applicable to the children's protocol, one dramatic difference between the two populations surfaced soon after centers began implanting children. This difference was in the critical area of postimplant habilitation.

Adults who received the implant responded well to postimplant training conducted in drill and practice type sessions in the hospital clinic after surgery. In fact, many of the listening activities, once introduced by the therapist in the clinic, were relegated to home practice by the client, or with a spouse or other companion. After a short period of listening practice, the adult developed many of the auditory skills that were now made possible by the implant. An adult was likely to be dismissed from therapy after a fixed period of time and seen subsequently only for the routine visits to set the device.

Children, on the other hand, were found to be a more heterogeneous group with regard to their language abilities prior to implantation and needed more extensive (re)habilitation. Potential candidates for the device presented with a range of ages (from 2 to 17 years), a continuum of language abilities (from no formal system to complex language competence), a number of communication systems (oral, cued speech, or total communication), and vastly different educational placements (residential school for the deaf to mainstream settings). No one training package could be designed to meet all these varied needs. Further, children who were among the first to be implanted often traveled great distances to the implant center. Participating in an extended training program at the hospital or clinic so far from home was impractical. This type of center-based model ignored the fact that the children seeking implants were likely enrolled in some kind of educational program to which they would return after implantation. Given the long-term commitment that schools make to their students, it seemed unwise to overlook their role in the implantation process. Centers interested in designing a protocol that would meet the vast needs of the young deaf child were forced to rethink candidacy selection issues, the design of their service delivery system for postimplant habilitation, and recruitment of additional personnel to provide the array of services required by the deaf child. These centers expanded their existing team for the process of implantation in children.

The concept of a multidisciplinary team approach to the management of children with hearing loss is not a new one (Matkin, Hook, & Hixson, 1979; Nevins, 1986). This often meant that the audiologist, school psychologist, speech-language pathologist, occupational and physical therapists, as well as the classroom teacher, each evaluated and developed a comprehensive educational plan for the hearing-impaired child. Cochlear implant technology necessitated a recasting of the concept of the team approach so that the team was now *inter*disciplinary rather than *multi*disciplinary and also included an otologic surgeon.

Because the insertion of the cochlear implant is a surgical procedure, a medical model of deafness is likely to drive the process of implantation. The medical model (see Chapter 1) suggests that deafness is a condition to be diagnosed and treated, in this case with a cochlear implant. However, unlike other forms of medical intervention (e.g., appendectomy, tonsillectomy, or conventional drug therapy) implantation is a process and not simply a treatment. It requires an extensive time commitment and a rarely seen partnership between the medical and educational communities. The application of the traditional medical model in cases of implantation may not be appropriate.

Physicians are assumed to be the "captain" of the team in traditional medical models. However, many surgeons may be unfamiliar with the educational needs of deaf children. Thus, what is needed is a truly collaborative team in which individuals take varied roles of equal importance, alternating in the position of "expert." This is in contrast to the traditional medical pyramid with a primary expert at the top and all else viewed as implementers. Team members should be able to explore their individual areas and make recommendations without pressures that view the surgery as a treatment end. Surgeons who are committed to the perspective of implantation as a process and not a treatment will embrace this team approach to the management of children with implants. Incorporating a team approach, however, is not without its problems.

■ CHARACTERISTICS OF MEDICAL AND EDUCATIONAL ENVIRONMENTS

Professionals in both hospitals and schools work under demanding time constraints that preclude easy access for communication with one another. The teacher cannot be called away from the classroom during class time; the itinerant is often in transit and simply unavailable. The physician's responsibilities to individual patient appointments and surgery leave little time during the teacher's school day for direct communication. Thus, creating a hospital/school communication link appears to be impossible.

Even if a communication link is created, individuals who have been in both hospitals and schools know that these are two vastly different environments. Although both the hospital and the school are structured to provide services in the best manner possible, there are certain inherent differences that may impede information exchange between and among professionals in each system. Chief among these differences is the language and vocabulary each uses to describe its function or treatment. Medical jargon is not well understood by the educator, nor is "educationalese" understood by the health care professional (and neither is understood by the parent).

Medical interaction is generally short term in nature and related to a crisis in health, whereas the educational environment lends itself to the establishment of more long-term relationships. Costs and methods of income retrieval for each of the systems also differ markedly. The hospital-based system provides billable and codable services which are paid directly by the consumer or reimbursed through third-party payers. Services are dispensed to individuals based on their specific needs. Educational costs, on the other hand, are broad and are not billed specifically. They are paid globally through property taxes or individually by the consumer through tuition. Services are dispensed to groups based on district-wide curriculum and rarely based on individual needs. The unique nature of the educational input required by students with implants makes it difficult for payment to be retrieved for this service, which is a medical/educational hybrid.

The differences between hospitals and schools, however, should not be viewed as irreconcilable. A child-centered team approach to cochlear implantation that includes both medical and educational personnel should support the cochlear implant process. A critical member of the implant team is the educator of the deaf who attempts to provide the necessary link between the hospital and school communities.

■ THE EDUCATIONAL CONSULTANT MODEL

The U.S. Food and Drug Administration (FDA) guidelines that regulate implant surgery do not dictate the presence of an educator on the implant team. The guidelines do suggest, however, that candidates for implants be enrolled in educational programs that emphasize auditory and speech skills. An educational consultant, working on a pediatric cochlear implant team, can ascertain whether a child's local school program is one that values listening and speaking. This individual is a certified teacher of the deaf with experience in the development of speech, spoken language, and auditory skills (Nevins, Kretschmer, Chute, Hellman, & Parisier, 1991). The presence of an educational consultant is a factor which can impact greatly upon the child's success with the implant.

There now exists an international organization known as The Network of Educators of Children with Cochlear Implants (NECCI).

This group comprises educators, speech-language pathologists, and educational audiologists in the United States, Canada, Europe, and Australia who have identified themselves as professionals committed to the process of implantation (see Appendix A for information regarding membership in NECCI). In 1994, a core group of NECCI members representative of a variety of backgrounds and geographical areas developed a position statement which supports the importance of the role of the educational consultant on a cochlear implant team. This position paper, seen in Figure 2–1 reflects the growing awareness of the contributions an educator can offer throughout the implant process.

■⃞ RESPONSIBILITIES OF THE EDUCATIONAL CONSULTANT

It is recommended that the educational consultant make an initial school visit *prior* to implantation as part of the evaluation for candidacy. The purpose of this preimplant visit is both fact finding and information dissemination (Nevins et al., 1991). The four basic goals of the preimplant school visit by the educational consultant are outlined in Table 2–1. The educational consultant arranges for the school visit soon after the child's first appointment at the implant center.

Because there is still much misinformation about implants and the process of implantation, it is important for the educational consultant to spend some time with school personnel to provide them with facts about the device in general and its potential benefit for the child. Often, questions from the child's teachers and other staff drive the nature and level of the information presented at this preimplant period. For instance, when a child is in a mainstream setting, questions about deafness and language development may be of greater concern to the child's teachers than is the difference between hearing aid and implant technology. The discussion regarding device technology may be of more interest to teachers of the deaf and speech-language pathologists.

Because the preimplant visit generally occurs after the speech and language evaluation has taken place at the implant center, the educational consultant can verify performance observed by the team's speech-language pathologist. It is not uncommon for young children to show greater communication ability in a more familiar school environment than in the hospital evaluation area. Because factors of speech and language ability affect candidacy decisions (see Chapter 4) it is important that the child's best performance level be obtained.

Network of Educators
of Children with Cochlear Implants
Position Statement

It is the position of the Network of Educators of Children with Cochlear Implants (NECCI) that:

1. Cochlear implants are a viable alternative for improving auditory skills in hearing-impaired children who receive little or no benefit from an intensive auditory program using more conventional amplification.

2. Medical and audiological factors should not be the exclusive criteria used in selecting candidates for implantation.

3. Cultural and educational factors are essential components which must be evaluated in selecting children who may benefit from the implant.

4. Best practice mandates that an educator who is knowledgeable about audition and auditory habilitation/rehabilitation be included as an essential member of the implant team during the entire implantation process, from evaluation and selection through habilitation/rehabilitation.

5. The educator is in the best position to:
   a. evaluate critical educational factors which affect the potential for success with the implant, and
   b. direct the necessary auditory habilitation/rehabilitation.

6. The educator can facilitate communication and cooperation among the family, medical facility, and educational settings, optimizing the child's potential for effective use of the implant.

7. The benefits derived from a cochlear implant are directly related to the habilitation/rehabilitation services provided in the child's post-implant educational program. Accordingly, an intensive, long-term program of auditory skill development should be seen as a critical component in the child's education.

Therefore, NECCI strongly recommends that parents considering an implant for their child seek out centers and educational settings that include an educator knowledgeable about appropriate habilitation/rehabilitation with the implant.

The above position statement was developed by members of the Network of Educators of Children with Cochlear Implants who were selected to participate in a THINK TANK held at the Manhattan Eye, Ear & Throat Hospital. THINK TANK participants represent educators, speech-language pathologists, audiologists, and auditory-verbal therapists from across the United States.

Figure 2–1
Network of Educators of Children with Cochlear Implants (NECCI) Position Statement. (From NECCI News 1992, reprinted with permission.)

TABLE 2–1

Goals and Related Activities of the Preimplant School Visit by the Educational Consultant.

Goals	Activities
To disseminate information about the implant cochlear implant	1. Distribute information about the cochlear implant device 2. Answer questions about candidacy, surgery, and how the implant works
To assess the educational environment of the candidate	1. Record placement type (residential, special class, mainstream) and availability of support services 2. Interview school administrators and personnel
To evaluate the child's performance in school environment	1. Observe child in classroom and in special activities (e.g., speech) 2. Examine relevant school records 3. Interview teachers and support personnel
To establish a working relationship between implant center and school	1. Encourage school personnel to voice opinion on child's candidacy for the implant 2. Create opportunities for informal exchange between local school staff and the Educational Consultant

Interviews with the teacher for impressions of the child and his over-all abilities are considered vitally important to the decision-making process. School personnel should be viewed as extended members of the implant team whose input is integral to evaluating candidacy.

In addition to observing children in classrooms and individual speech therapy settings, the educational consultants assess the overall educational environment of the school program. Consultants will identify the placement as residential, day school, self-contained day class, resource room, or mainstream. This information will affect the nature and extent of the knowledge and skill that staff will need to acquire to accomplish postimplant goals. The educational consultants may also meet with school administrators to determine the availability of support services for children following implant surgery.

■□ ESTABLISHING A WORKING RELATIONSHIP

Despite the importance of all of the activities already listed in the preimplant visit of the educational consultant, the single most important objective of this visit is the establishment of a trusting relationship between the implant center and the school. If the child is indeed deemed a candidate and receives an implant, the school should, in most cases, be given the lead role in providing habilitation after surgery. The work of maximizing the effects of the auditory information available through the device will be the responsibility of the local school personnel. Unlike adults who return to the implant center for drill and practice with the implant, the child returns to his local school for long-term education. It would be wise to enlist the aid of these professionals in providing the necessary habilitation services. The educational consultant will determine the level of information and training required by local personnel to design postimplant habilitation.

In some cases, the school personnel may be knowledgeable about the development of auditory skills with traditional amplification but have had no experience with children with cochlear implants. In these circumstances, the educational consultant will provide information about the implant device and how it works so as to combat fear of the unknown technology. Simultaneously, the educational consultant will reinforce the staff's ability to provide for auditory activities in the classroom. In still other cases, the staff may be unfamiliar with the device but also be uncertain about how to develop auditory skills. When school-based personnel are open to guidance from the educational consultant, it is necessary to offer it in the proper spirit. We believe that spirit to be one of collegial collaboration, not one that is either overly simplistic or pedantic in nature. The seeds of what will be a long-term partnership must be planted at the time of the preimplant visit. The tone set by the educational consultant will influence the nature of that partnership that will again be important during postimplant follow up.

■□ THE POSTIMPLANT PHASE

Once the device has been implanted and the surgical incision has healed, the child is seen for stimulation of the device. If possible, the educational consultant attends these device setting sessions to observe the child's first responses to sound. It is important for the educational consultant to be knowledgeable of the exact level of performance demonstrated by the child at the time of the initial device activation so that recommendations for introductory teaching objectives can be made to local school personnel. After identifying these objectives (see Chapter 6), the educational consultant allows the local school personnel time to familiarize themselves with the device, observe the child's response to sound in the school environment, and develop questions. Thus, a follow-up visit is not scheduled until approximately 4 weeks after the initial stimulation of the device.

■□ TRAINING FOR CARE AND MANAGEMENT OF THE DEVICE

During the postimplant visit, the educational consultant reviews issues regarding the care and management of the device; specifically, teachers are shown techniques for performing daily equipment checks. Although some level of equipment check can be performed independently of the child, the daily check should also include a measure of the child's auditory performance once he is capable of responding. For example, the teacher may request the child to raise his hand after each auditory-only presentation of the six sound test (ah, ee, oo, s, sh, m) (Perigoe, 1992). As the child's skill with the implant increases, listening check tasks can be made more difficult. A child with advanced skills may be given a topic, and the teacher will name items appropriate to that topic. In this case, the teacher may tell the child that the topic is animals and say "dog," "horse," "bird," "cat," and "fish." Despite the fact that parents are performing listening checks at home, the teacher should perform a listening check at school to ensure that the child has a functioning device throughout the day. Should teachers discover that the device is not functioning properly, they must implement techniques to correct the problem. It is the responsibility of the educational consultant to provide teachers with this knowledge and how to troubleshoot the device. (More detailed information on care and management of the device and troubleshooting techniques can be found in Chapter 6.)

■□ DIRECTING THE ESTABLISHMENT OF APPROPRIATE AUDITORY GOALS

The educational consultant also offers guidance to the teacher/therapist regarding the importance of providing an environment that facilitates auditory learning (see Chapter 7), while simultaneously acknowledging the demands and the realities of a school day. The educational consultant's postimplant visit again requires observation in the classroom and therapy settings so that specific recommendations about incorporating listening in these environments can be made. This observation enables the educational consultant to become familiar with a particular classroom's routine, and use real-life examples to identify opportunities that maximize listening.

An additional function of the educational consultant is to provide input into the development of the child's Individualized Educational Plan (IEP). As the on-site expert in cochlear implant technology and habilitation, the educational consultant can enumerate goals and objectives in the area of auditory skill development that are child and device specific. In some instances, local school personnel may not have the background knowledge to design a comprehensive speech and language program for the child with an implant. This is often the case when children are in rural areas where there are no other deaf children or are in mainstream environments. Frequently, the educational consultant will make recommendations regarding speech and language goals in addition to auditory goals in order to provide this necessary component to the child's total plan.

■□ LONG-TERM FOLLOW-UP

Issues of educational management of the child with an implant do not end at any specified time after the child receives the device. Rather, they grow and change as the child moves through the educational system. The child's needs dictate the role of the educational consultant and the emphasis she places on the many aspects of total development. At the time of implantation, issues of auditory learning may be of paramount importance. Subsequent success with the device may cause previously overshadowed problems to surface. For example, a profoundly deaf child achieving good auditory and speech skills may find his way into a mainstream classroom. There, general problems with learning may be detected as the pace of instruction is increased when compared to the careful and methodical teaching that generally occurs in the self-contained classroom. Failure to address a learning problem that is observed later in the child's educational career may jeopardize past accomplishments made possible by the implant. The continued involvement of the educational consultant during the period of long-term follow-up ensures that the appropriate services will be available to the child throughout his school years. This involvement will dictate an ongoing commitment on the part of the implant facility to a child-centered approach to the process of implantation.

■□ SUMMARY

Cochlear implantation is a process, not simply a treatment for deafness. It requires a team of professionals committed to the long-term care of the children who receive the device. Because part of that long-term care occurs simultaneously with the education of the child, it is logical that school-based professionals are included as extended members of the implant team. It is the implant center's educational consultant who is charged with the task of enlisting the aid of local school personnel. Although it is the surgeon who assumes the lead role in the initial stages of the process of implantation by performing the surgery, the educational consultant is the individual who continues the process throughout the child's educational career. Facilities which do not address educational issues of children with implants may find the responsibility of their management during the postimplant phase overwhelming.

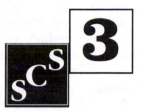

History, Development, and Current Technology

Technological advances in the United States are a cooperative effort among manufacturers, laboratories, and consumers. This process is carefully regulated and controlled by governmental agencies that oversee the stages of development in order to protect the general population. These controls govern the industries which manufacture both drugs and technology, which eventually become available to the public. There are times when the presence of the FDA is considered a nuisance; however, its existence prevents the premature introduction of products without supervised study.

■□ THE FDA PROCESS

Before examining the history of cochlear implants, it is important to understand the FDA process through which all medical devices in the United States have passed. The initial development of any device usually begins in one laboratory under the auspices of a principle investigator. At this stage, a small number of subjects receive the new technology and are carefully followed. In all cases, the population under study consists of adults who are capable of giving full consent for their participation. This period is considered to be the experimental stage and represents the earliest phase of development for any device.

After preliminary data are gathered on a small subgroup of the population to monitor both the safety and efficacy of the device, a report is made to the FDA to apply for investigational status. Investigational status will permit a predetermined number of facilities across the United States to perform similar tests on a designated group of subjects who meet specified criteria for selection. This is done for two reasons: first, to demonstrate that the results obtained by the principle investigator are replicable by other laboratories, and second, to accrue more subjects in a timely fashion across a widespread population base.

Once a larger subject base has been amassed and studied for a time period longer than the experimental phase, the results are again reported to the FDA with a request for premarket approval. Premarket approval enables the technology to be made available to any center interested in clinically using the device. Generally, it is at this stage or just prior to it that studies in children or other subpopulations are permitted. Subjects identified during the original investigational stage continue to be monitored to observe any possible changes in device-related effects.

The premarket stage continues until the government grants final full-market approval. When final full-market approval is achieved no further data collection is necessary. Presently, data continue to be collected to monitor long-term benefits of the implant. Although several cochlear implant devices have obtained premarket approval in this country, to date, no implant has received final full-market approval. The practical differences, however, between premarket approval and full-market approval are negligible to the consumer because, under both conditions, the device is freely available.

■□ THE COCHLEAR IMPLANT SYSTEM

All cochlear implants have similar features. Every system consists of a surgically implanted portion and a set of external components. The implanted segment consists of either one or several electrodes and circuitry to deliver the signal. These electrodes are, in most cases, implanted into the scala tympani of the cochlea (see Figure 3–1, cross section of cochlea).

The external components consist of a microphone, speech processor, transmitter, and cords. Incoming signals are detected by the

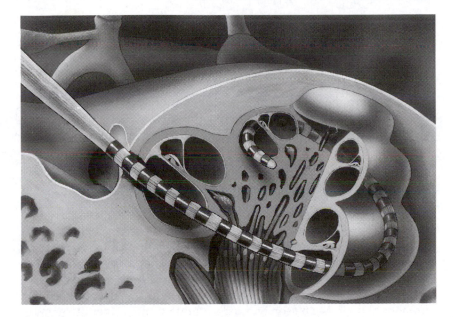

Figure 3–1
Cross section of cochlea showing the placement of the electrode in the scala tympani. (Photograph courtesy of Cochlear Corporation.)

microphone and delivered to the speech processor through a cord which connects the two pieces of equipment. The speech processor then converts that information into a code that is individual to each of the systems. This information is sent back up to the external transmitter where it is then delivered to the internal receiver either by magnetic induction or direct connection. Several electrodes or, in some cases, only one electrode are activated based on a program that is individual to the device. Electrodes transmit the electrical signals to residual auditory nerve fibers in the cochlea which carry them to the brain for interpretation. The difference between devices is in the manner the signal is processed and the number of electrodes stimulated. A brief history and review of the systems that have been or are being used in the pediatric population follows.

■□ THE HISTORY OF COCHLEAR IMPLANTS

One of the first attempts at electrical stimulation of the cochlea was performed in France in 1957 by Djourno and Eyries. During stapes surgery, gold electrodes were placed on the promontory (located between the round window and oval window) of the cochlea and an electrical current was delivered across the surgical field. The patient, who was under local anesthesia and awake, reported hearing a sound during this procedure. This attempt at auditory stimulation through electrical excitation remained an obscure notation in medical journals until the late 1960s. At that time, Dr. William House, in Los Angeles, California, along with an electronics engineer named Jack Urban, became intrigued with the work of the French surgeons and attempted to develop a clinically applicable system of cochlear stimulation. Simultaneously, Dr. Robin Michelson, in San Francisco, California, and Dr. Blair Simmons at Stanford also began work in this area. Although Dr. House implanted a multielectrode system, he concentrated his work on a single electrode device. In the meantime, both Dr. Simmons and Dr. Michelson worked separately and diligently on multiple electrode stimulation in an effort to mimic the normal cochlea. Since the normal auditory system consists of a great number of functioning hair cells distributed throughout the cochlea, multiple sites of stimulation would be more representative of the incoming signal than a single point. It was believed that any attempt at artificially stimulating the neural elements remaining in deafened cochleas was best accomplished at numerous locations. In later years, Dr. Robert Schindler, at the University of California at San Francisco, continued the research in the area of multichannel stimulation pioneered by Dr. Michelson (House & Berliner, 1991).

Meanwhile, Dr. House persisted with his efforts to develop a wearable cochlear implant using single channel stimulation. This device consisted of one ball electrode and transmitted speech through a processor with only one channel. The initial studies, which focused on safety and efficacy issues, commenced in adults in the 1970s (House & Urban, 1973). During the investigational phase of the study, only seven centers in the United States were granted permission by the FDA to implant this device in adults who were profoundly deaf. Early protocols included an extensive battery of both audiological and psychological tests. Routine evaluations were performed to monitor the auditory changes that occurred with implant use and also to ensure that there was no deleterious effect from the electrical stimulation.

The early version of the 3M/House device was known as the Sigma 6 or Sigma 7 and used transcutaneous (across the skin) coupling. The external transmitter was held in place through an elaborate arrangement which used a headband or eyeglasses with a cuplike extension in which the transmitter was held (see Figure 3–2). Obviously, slippage of the headband or the eyeglasses resulted in a loss of electrical transmission. The speech processor was large (the dimensions of the Sigma 7 were 5 × 2½ × 1 inch), encased in metal, and powered by two 9-volt batteries which required replacement after approximately 40–80 hours of use. Despite the cumbersome cosmetics of the device, individuals who used it were enthusiastic.

Skepticism within the medical community about the use of this device surfaced due to the lack of controlled studies and the claim of benefit based on anecdotal reports. However, in 1977, an independent study by Bilger et al. (1977) was undertaken. A series of adults who had been implanted with the single channel system were evaluated with a variety of speech perception and speechreading measures. Bilger and

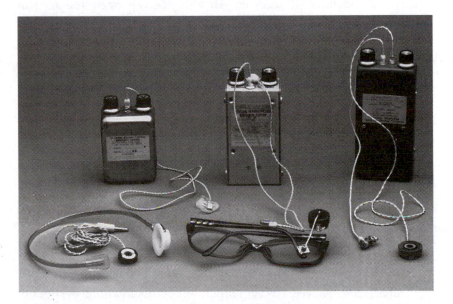

Figure 3–2
Early version of single channel devices. (Photograph courtesy of House Ear Institute.)

his associates found that all the subjects could detect pure tone signals and speech at approximately 40 dB HTL when using their implants. In addition, many were able to detect the timing and intensity cues in ongoing speech. However, none was able to understand speech without the aid of visual cues. Although the majority of the adults demonstrated some improvement in their ability to speechread when their device was activated, some exhibited no effect. Additionally, many subjects demonstrated a ceiling effect during this evaluation; performance was at a maximum in the vision-alone condition and therefore the vision-plus-audition condition yielded little measurable enhancement. Nonetheless, all subjects reported improved "quality of life" that fostered continued use of the device.

Breakthrough Technology

The pace of implantation was progressing slowly when, in 1980, Dr. Jack Hough, in Oklahoma City, Oklahoma, developed a rare earth magnet that could be surgically implanted without creating interference with the internal receiver. This magnet changed the face of implantation drastically by making transmission across the skin more precise and less variable between and within subjects. With one magnet implanted internally and one placed externally in the transmitter, implant users were able to make a more direct and stable connection between the two portions of the device. This eliminated the use of the cumbersome external gadgets which held the transmitter in place and were only mildly successful. The development of the magnet paved the way for the implantation of the device in children. Prior to the magnet's introduction, one of the concerns regarding implantation in children was related to the ability of the device to maintain a consistent signal to the child.

As the magnet was being introduced, the 3M Corporation began its involvement with the House device. With support from 3M, much of the manufacturing of the device moved from the laboratories at the House Ear Institute into the mainstream of the corporate world. The financial and technical backing that was necessary to allow the cochlear implant program to expand and maintain service was made available by 3M. Unfortunately, years later, corporate decisions would eventually lead to the withdrawal of the company from the implant industry.

Initial Results with Single Channel Implants

A total of 269 adults received the single channel cochlear implant during the period of clinical trials (Thielemeir, 1985). Interestingly, the initial studies on implanted adults pooled all subjects together regardless of age of onset of deafness. This resulted in the reporting of the abilities of prelinguistically deafened adults and postlinguistically deafened adults together. Subsequent studies have demonstrated that these two groups of subjects perform differently. Combining the data for each of the subgroups lowered the overall group performance with the device. Future studies involving other implant devices would separate these two categories to make certain that the results were indicative of the specific population.

In November 1983, the 3M/House device received premarket approval from the FDA for use in the adult population. Trials had already begun in California to determine the safety and efficacy of using this device in children. Late in 1983, the FDA granted an investigational device exemption for the same seven centers that had taken part in the adult clinical trials to proceed with implanting children. Table 3–1 lists the names and locations of these first implantation centers.

TABLE 3–1
Listing of Eight Original Co-Investigators of the 3M/House Cochlear Implant System.

House Ear Institute Los Angeles, California Dr. William House	Baptist Medical Center Oklahoma City, Oklahoma Dr. Jack Hough
Denver Ear Institute Denver, Colorado Dr. Thomas Balkany	Midwest Ear Institute Kansas City, Missouri Dr. Charles Leutje
Indiana University Indianapolis, Indiana Dr. Richard Miyamoto	Texas Ear Institute Dallas, Texas Dr. Ed Maddox
Cleveland Clinic Cleveland, Ohio Dr. Sam Kinney	Manhattan Eye, Ear & Throat Hospital New York, New York Dr. Simon Parisier

Clinical trials ended several years later without premarket approval ever having been granted to the 3M/House device for children. This occurred partly as a result of the 3M Corporation's disinterest in remaining in the cochlear implant market and the more impressive results observed with the multichannel Nucleus device. When the rights to the 3M/House device were sold to Cochlear Corporation (the manufacturer of the Nucleus device), the fate of the single channel was all but sealed.

During the same time period, work on a multielectrode, multichannel implant continued at the University of California at San Francisco (UCSF) under the direction of Drs. Schindler and Michelson. This device was promising in that it offered finer detail regarding pitch discrimination, but the packaging of the internal receiver was extremely large. In Australia, the Nucleus Corporation had already begun clinical studies into the use of a multichannel system (Clark, 1987). This device, known as the Nucleus 22 channel cochlear implant system, was being studied in groups of deaf adults both in the United States and in Australia. The performance of subjects using the multichannel devices was encouraging because many of the adult users were capable of understanding some speech without the aid of visual cues.

Although multichannel stimulation provided information regarding the durational aspects of speech, it offered more details about pitch. Stimulation at multiple electrode sites within the cochlea permitted the presentation of different channels of information. The term *channels* indicates the number of electrode sites which convey different information. Stimulation over numerous channels enabled the signal to be divided into certain components so that it could be processed and delivered in a more exact manner. Hence, the amount and nature of the information which was transferred to the cochlea was greatly improved. These additional cues contributed to better performance overall. Although there were several multichannel implants under study at this time, the Nucleus device was the first to offer a clinically usable implant which had widespread appeal.

In 1984, the FDA granted premarket approval status for use of the Nucleus device in the postlinguistically deafened adult population. Shortly after, clinical trials in children began in the United States. With the superiority of performance that was evident from the Nucleus device, coupled with the realization that the market for the cochlear implant was relatively small, the 3M Corporation decided to remove itself from the implant business. Cochlear Corporation (the American subsidiary of Nucleus) then purchased the 3M/House device in order to provide service for those children and adults who were implanted with it. These services are still maintained by Cochlear Corporation today.

The investigation into the safety and efficacy of the Nucleus device included 142 children who were implanted by 36 centers in the United States and abroad (Staller, Dowell, Beiter, & Brimacombe, 1991). The majority of these children were followed for at least 2 years. The results of this study documented the improvement in performance on a variety of speech perception tasks evaluated in these children (see Chapter 11). In 1989, the FDA granted premarket approval for the use of the Nucleus 22 channel cochlear implant system in children between the ages of 2 through 17 years. To date, it is the only cochlear implant system to have received premarket approval for use in both adults and children. The Nucleus 22 channel implant represents the cochlear implant system with the largest number of users (10,000 adults and children) in the world (Cochlear Corporation, personal communication, January, 1995).

Despite the momentum behind the Nucleus device, two other research groups continued to work in the United States in the implant field. One group, located in Utah, was investigating a multichannel system known initially as the Symbion device, and later the Ineraid. Although the Ineraid was part of an adult clinical trials protocol in the United States, it still has not received premarket approval from the FDA. The device has never been used in the pediatric population in this country. A second group at the University of California at San Francisco (UCSF) continued its work in the area of multichannel signal processing. The investigators at UCSF took another decade of research before finally developing a usable clinical system. This device, now known as the Clarion, is completing its clinical trials in the adult population and beginning studies in children.

Although cochlear implant systems may vary depending on the number of electrodes that are implanted or the number of channels that process the signal, the method of (re)habilitation remains similar. The cochlear implant should be viewed as a tool which enables its user to obtain functional information about the speech signal. The utility of this information can be maximized and enhanced through practice. This practice can be short term (as demonstrated by many of the adult cochlear implant users) or continue over years of implant use (as observed with the pediatric population). The importance of postimplant (re)habilitation for children receiving cochlear implants remains the most critical factor in maximizing the benefit from the device.

■▢ PAST AND CURRENT DEVICES IMPLANTED IN CHILDREN

Two devices, the 3M/House and the Nucleus 22 channel implant, have been used in the pediatric population in the United States. A third device, the Clarion, has begun clinical trials for this group. As previously noted, there are a number of features similar to all cochlear implant system. Specific information for each device follows.

The 3M/House Cochlear Implant System

The 3M/House device was originally named the House system in honor of its inventor, Dr. William House. When 3M Corporation became involved in its financing and marketing, the name was changed to the 3M/House cochlear implant. The implant's internal components consist of a single ball electrode and an internal receiver. Also encased in the internal receiver is a magnet to allow easy alignment with the external components. Externally, a microphone, which can be worn either on an earhook or on the lapel, is connected by a cord to the speech processor. A second cord connects the speech processor to the external transmitter. This external transmitter also contains a magnet which creates the connection to the implanted device. Information is transmitted through the skin to the single ball electrode that has been implanted approximately 6 mm into the cochlea.

Speech Processing Strategy

The 3M/House cochlear implant system uses a relatively simple form of speech processing. The analog waveform (i.e., the representation of the whole wave) of the speech is amplified, filtered, and modulated using a 16k Hz tone. The amplifier increases the overall strength of the signal, while the filter determines which frequencies will be delivered or rejected. The modulation tone is used to prevent the signal from sounding like noise. This information is then delivered to the single ball electrode located in the cochlea. Information in the speech signal which characterizes the timing and intensity cues are transmitted best. Selective frequency information is not represented because the processor does not extract this information. The entire signal is delivered to only one electrode.

The Nucleus 22 Channel Cochlear Implant System

This system was developed in Australia at the University of Melbourne under the direction of Dr. Graeme Clark (Clark, 1987) and is manufactured in the United States by Cochlear Corporation in Colorado. The implanted receiver-stimulator consists of sophisticated circuitry, a magnet, and an electrode array made up of 22 platinum bands. This electrode array is inserted approximately 25 mm into the scala tympani. Externally, a microphone, which is packaged in a traditional behind-the-ear hearing aid case, is connected via a cord to the speech processor and to the external transmitter (see Figure 3–3).

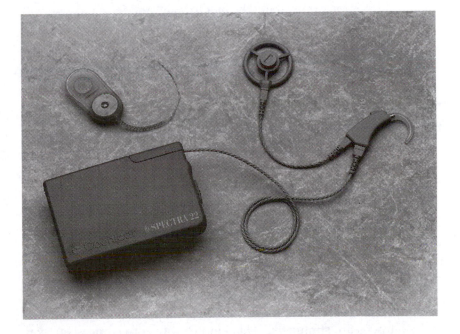

Figure 3–3
Nucleus 22 Channel Cochlear Implant System. (Photograph courtesy of Cochlear Corporation.)

Speech-Processing Strategies

The speech-processing strategy used by the Nucleus device has changed significantly over the past several years. The initial processor known as the Wearable Speech Processor (WSP) incorporated a feature extractor that selected certain characteristics of the speech signal to present to the electrode array in the cochlea. These were the fundamental frequency, amplitude, and the second formant. These features were chosen because they provided a relatively good representation of the speech signal. The fundamental frequency was coded as the pulse rate, and the second formant information determined which electrode would be stimulated. Amplitude was coded by the current level used to stimulate the electrodes. Initial studies with this device demonstrated good benefit (Dowell, Mecklenburg, & Clark, 1986); however, the addition of information which represented the first formant was found to increase speech discrimination further (Dowell, Seligman, Blamey, & Clark, 1987). This later generation of the WSP (known as the WSP III) included information about the first formant and required a second electrode to be activated during the signal processing.

Research into the development of better signal processing schemes continued and in 1989, another generation of the Nucleus device known as the Mini Speech Processor (MSP) became available. With the introduction of the MSP, the physical size of the speech processor was reduced and a new speech strategy was incorporated. This strategy known as Multipeak (MPEAK) delivered supplementary high frequency information to the cochlea. In addition to the fundamental frequency, first formant, and second formant, three high frequency bands were added (Patrick & Clark, 1991). Results with this strategy indicated marked improvement over the WSP III (Skinner et al., 1991).

In April 1994, yet another speech processor and strategy was introduced. This processor, the Spectra 22, incorporated a new type of speech strategy known as Spectral Peak (SPEAK). SPEAK was developed after several years of research in Australia which indicated improved performance with this processing variation (McKay & McDermott, 1991). This latest advance abandoned the feature extractor scheme; it analyzes the whole speech waveform and identifies the six maximal peaks of the waveform. These six peaks determine which six electrodes are stimulated. This kind of waveform processing was believed to deliver more information about the speech waveform and thus provide better discrimination. Although this strategy is relatively new, studies in adults in the United States, (Skinner, Forakis, Holden,

& Holden, 1994) and children in Australia (Cowan et al., 1994) indicate better performance especially in background noise.

The Clarion Cochlear Implant System

The Clarion device, manufactured by Advanced Bionics Corporation, located in Sylmar, California, is the latest manufacturer to enter the adult and pediatric cochlear implant market in the United States. This device was developed after years of work at the University of California at San Francisco. There are substantial differences both internally and externally between this multichannel device and the Nucleus 22 channel implant. The internal portion which is surgically implanted contains 16 ball electrodes situated in pairs around the array. Eight of these are located medially and eight laterally. The electrode array itself is precoiled and resembles a pig's tail in order to provide more efficient electrical stimulation closer to the neural tissue.

The device is packaged in a ceramic case which also includes a magnet to hold the device on the head. Externally, a transmitter, with a recessed microphone is worn. With the microphone housed directly in the external transmitter, an additional piece of hardware on the head is not required as it is with the Nucleus device. The headset is also capable of providing bidirectional telemetry. Bidirectional telemetry enables the clinician to measure electrical information (i.e., impedances) directly from the implanted internal receiver. It provides the clinician with a quick and easy method of determining the functioning of the internal device. Like the Nucleus, the external transmitter is connected to the speech processor via a cord. The complete Clarion system is illustrated in Figure 3–4.

Speech-Processing Strategies

The Clarion speech processor differs from the Nucleus device in several ways. The Clarion processor can be programmed to retain more than one speech-processing formula. This multistrategy approach offers the user a choice of programs throughout the day. The types of speech-processing strategies which can be programmed are also different from the Nucleus. The first of these strategies is known as Continuous Interleaved Sampling (CIS) and provides a rapid sampling technique to deliver the signal in a sequence of a large number

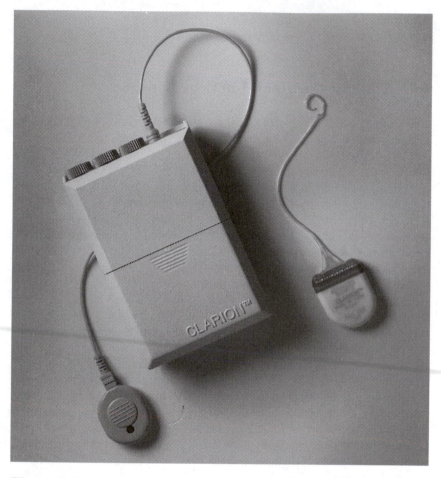

Figure 3–4
Complete Clarion Multi-Strategy Cochlear Implant System. (Photograph courtesy of Advanced Bionics Corporation.)

of pulses to the implanted electrodes (Wilson, 1993). By interleaving pulses, stimulation is cycled through the electrode array thereby providing nonsimultaneous stimulation. The implanted electrodes can be programmed in a variety of ways to maximize the individual's residual auditory capabilities. A second type of speech-processing strategy known as Compressed Analog (CA) is also available. The major difference between CA and CIS is that CA presents continuous analog signals, whereas CIS presents pulses. Some cochlear implant recipients use both strategies under different listening conditions (e.g., for music or in noise), whereas others have a preference for just one of the speech strategies.

Although this device has only been available for postlinguistically deafened adults, clinical studies have recently begun with children. To accommodate its use in children, the physical size of the speech processor used for the adult clinical trials has been made substantially smaller. Average performance on a variety of speech perception measures has demonstrated better results than the MSP (Gantz, Tyler, Lowder, & Woodworth, 1995; Kessler, Zilberman, Roff, & Loeb, 1994). Although there are no data available for children with this device at the present time, the process of patient accrual began in June 1995, after permission from the FDA was granted.

■□ THE SURGERY

The surgical technique used for cochlear implantation is similar regardless of the device chosen. Although there are minor differences which occur between surgeons that are related to the size and shape of the incision, the basic procedure remains the same (Clark, Cohen, & Shepherd, 1991). The hair behind the ear of implantation is shaved and an incision is made. A skin flap (see Figure 3–5) is raised to expose the mastoid bone. A mastoidectomy (drilling of the mastoid bone) using a facial recess approach (identifying and using as a landmark the facial nerve) is used to approach the cochlea (see Figure 3–6). The electrode array is inserted into the scala tympani which is located beyond the round window membrane of the cochlea. For the Nucleus and 3M/House device, this array is slowly pushed into the scala tympani using a special fork-like tool (see Figure 3–7). Because the Clarion device is precoiled, it must be straightened at the time of the insertion. This is done through the use of a special insertion tool developed for this purpose (see Figure 3–8). Once the Clarion is inserted, the insertion tool is removed and the array retains its precoiled shape (Parisier, Chute, & Nevins, 1994).

In most cases, the electrode array is tied in place with special materials (Dacron) so that it will not extrude from the cochlea. The external transmitter portion of the array (i.e., the portion which houses the electronics of the device and the magnet) is placed on the temporal bone. This bone is smoothed down, and a bed the size of the

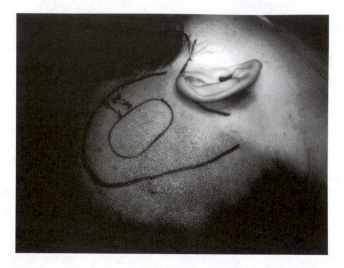

Figure 3–5
Patient preparation for surgery illustrating shaved head with markings
for incision. (Photograph courtesy of Mosby.)

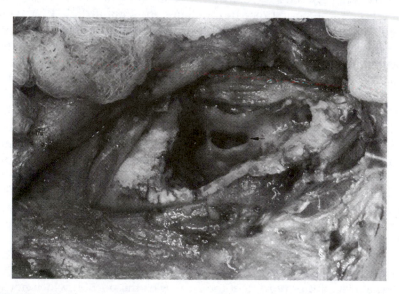

Figure 3–6
View of surgical approach to cochlea. (Photograph courtesy of Mosby.)

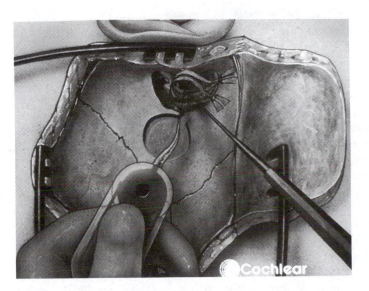

Figure 3-7
View of electrode being inserted into the cochlea. (Photograph courtesy of Cochlear Corporation.)

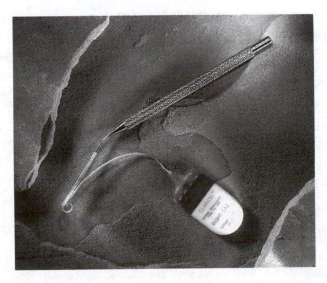

Figure 3-8
Clarion Multi-Strategy Insertion Tool. (Photograph courtesy of Advanced Bionics Corporation.)

receiver is drilled out. Small tunnels are made in the bone through which sutures are passed. These sutures are used to tied down the receiver so that it will not move around once the surgery has been completed (see Figure 3–9).

For very young children, a bed is not drilled out; the device is held in place using the muscles of the skull which are tied to encase it. The skin flap is closed using subcutaneous (under the skin) dissolvable sutures. The flap is held in place using regular sutures, staples or, in many cases with children, stirry strips (i.e., surgical tape). Some surgeons may insert a hemovac drain (small tube connected to a suction apparatus) which is removed before the child leaves the hospital. This is done to remove any fluid build up at the surgical site. In all cases, a large pressure bandage is placed over the wound to help keep swelling to a minimum.

The surgery, most often, is completed in 2–3 hours. The duration of the hospital stay will vary; it may be as short as 1 day in some hospitals and as long as 4 days in others. Generally, the child is admitted the morning of the surgery, is retained the day after surgery, and

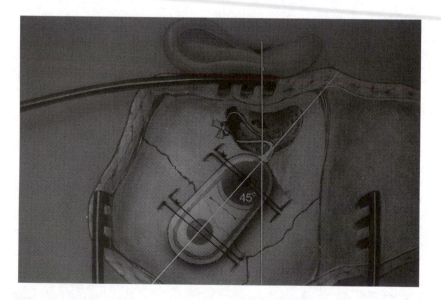

Figure 3–9
View of internal receiver sutured in place. (Photograph courtesy of Mosby.)

leaves the hospital on the morning of the third day. In a small percentage of cases, children may be nauseous and vomit immediately postoperatively. This is often a result of the general anesthesia and will pass rapidly and without consequence. When the implant recipient is ready to be discharged, he leaves the hospital with the bandage on. In some circumstance (especially in teenagers), the bandage is removed prior to leaving.

Approximately 1 week to 10 days after surgery, the implant recipient returns to the surgeon for a follow-up visit. During that period, the individual may not wash his hair. There are some parents who choose to keep their children home from school during this time. This is done more as a safety measure than as a medical necessity. In the majority of cases, children are able to resume normal activity almost immediately. With small children, who may be very active, precautions should be taken to ensure there is no trauma to the surgical site. Generally, the postoperative course is uneventful.

As the wound begins to heal, it will often itch. A child may scratch at the stirry strips (which, in most cases, fall off on their own) and create a scab. This is generally of no consequence, and the parents are instructed to use standard ointment (e.g., bacitracin or a cortisone cream) to control the problem. The most important issue at this time, especially for young active children, is to protect the child from picking at or injuring the area of the surgery. Many parents will restrict their child's activity during this initial healing period. Once the child returns to school, the parent may request that the child refrain from participating in physical education and other sports until the time of the initial stimulation. After the child is fully healed, he returns to the full complement of activity he enjoyed prior to implantation. Although there are some restrictions following cochlear implant surgery (see Chapter 6) these are fairly limited.

Postoperative Follow-Up

Careful postoperative follow up with specific attention to the surgical site should prevent problems from arising. Parents of children who have undergone surgery should be well informed about postoperative care. After the child has received the external equipment, the area under the external magnet should be routinely observed to ensure there is no undue pressure. Excessive pressure build up under the magnet will create an obvious depression which is extremely red in color. If this remains unchecked, there is a possibility that the skin in the area will thin and eventually erode, thereby exposing the internal portion of the implant. Generally, this will not occur. If an irritation of the area, with subsequent depression is noticed, the magnet strength should be reduced. When the lowest magnet strength is already in use, then a material known as Mole Skin can be purchased in the local pharmacy and placed over the magnet. Over time, these irritations heal without repercussion.

In addition to the area under the magnet, the general condition of the incision should be observed. On some occasions, there may be a subcutaneous suture which has not dissolved. This should not be removed by the parent. If a suture is noticed exiting the wound, the child should be seen by the surgeon for its extraction. Again, this is generally a simple procedure. It has no negative connotation regarding the outcome of the surgery.

The child should be seen regularly by the pediatrician, and, if an ear infection should occur, the implant surgeon should be informed. The presence of swelling in the area of the mastoid concomitant with a severe ear infection requires that the implanting surgeon be notified immediately. In most cases, ear infections resolve with standard antibiotic treatment. However, in cases in which they are unresponsive to traditional therapy, it is best for the child to return to the implanting surgeon for consultation. After implantation, the child should be seen yearly by the otologic surgeon who performed the surgery.

■□ THE FUTURE OF COCHLEAR IMPLANTS

The desire by implant users for a smaller speech processor is second only to the wish for better understanding through a cochlear implant. Although miniaturization of the external portions of the device is often considered secondary to the improvements in speech processing, it nonetheless remains a goal of the implant manufacturers. Unfortunately, the constraints imposed by battery technology may delay this process. As the sophistication of speech-processing strategies increases, so does the need for more electrical current. Until battery technology changes so that adequate power can be sent to newer, more-advanced microchips, progress in this area will remain stalled. Research and development continues to be focused on obtaining the best speech recognition possible for all hearing-impaired individuals as opposed to reducing the physical size of the device. Advances occurring over the past 5 years in the field of cochlear implants make it apparent that the issues of both speech processing and device size will be addressed and that the future of this technology is a promising one.

■□ SUMMARY

The rapid evolution of the cochlear implant from the early days of the simple, single channel device to the present day, sophisticated, multichannel systems has been fueled by the success of this technology. The cooperative efforts among manufacturers, medical facilities, and research laboratories throughout the United States have resulted in major advances in this field in a relatively short period of time. Today's implants are capable of transmitting more information of better quality so that device users have greater access to speech stimuli. Future technology is focused on improving processing capabilities further with an eventual reduction of the physical size of the device. Continued cooperation among medical and technological professionals will accelerate changes in this rapidly evolving field.

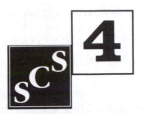

Pediatric Cochlear Implant Candidacy

The selection of appropriate candidates for cochlear implants is critical to the success of these devices in the pediatric population. Because children receiving cochlear implants will ultimately return to their local schools, the role of the classroom teacher is fundamental to the selection process. Unfortunately, teachers view themselves as passive in this process rather than being a primary information and/or referral source. To claim a more active role, teachers and speech and hearing professionals must become knowledgeable in all nuances of the selection process.

■□ GENERAL SELECTION CRITERIA

Historically, candidacy selection was vague and ill-defined. According to Berliner & Eisenberg (1985) the selection of candidates during the early phases of implant study centered around finding "good" subjects. These were individuals who lived locally and could make substantial time commitments. In later stages of implant investigation, the availability of regional centers made it possible for candidates to come from more diverse geographic areas. However, it was likely that these candidates would travel a great distance to a center for implant evaluation and follow-up.

Currently, the FDA has approved the following criteria for patient selection for the pediatric population:

1. Bilateral profound sensorineural deafness
2. Candidate age of 2 through 17 years
3. Little or no benefit from a hearing aid.

Further, no medical contraindications may be present, and families and candidates should be well motivated and possess appropriate expectations.

These stated criteria outline factors that are considered minimal requirements by many centers. If one looks more closely at these standards, however, a number of more subtle issues are left unstated. For example, "little or no benefit from a hearing aid" entails subjective interpretation. These judgments may differ depending on the professionals making decisions and the listening contexts in which they are made. For example, performance in the test setting may be different from that in real life or the classroom listening environment. Assessment of hearing aid benefit in only the clinical setting may provide insufficient information. The effectiveness of hearing aid use requires comprehensive inquiry prior to a decision to implant.

Centers with experience in implanting children have identified a number of additional issues that are evaluated in candidacy selection including speech and language abilities, cognitive and social readiness, and educational setting (Osberger et al., 1991a). Osberger et al. (1991a) have suggested that the primary question regarding implant candidacy has shifted from *if* the child is a candidate to *when* the child is a candidate. Answering the question of *when* the child is a candidate requires a cooperative effort between implant center and the child's long-term service providers. A growing number of implant centers recognize the important contribution that local school personnel play in providing information helpful to the implant team in choosing appropriate candidates (Nevins et al., 1991).

When teachers and speech-language pathologists are informed about all issues in candidate selection, they can become empowered to take an active rather than passive role as a child begins the evaluation procedure for implantation. Local school professionals generally have long-term knowledge of the child and his abilities and can provide valuable information to assist the implant team in making an informed candidacy decision. Unless teachers seek an active role in the preimplant process, they may be all but eliminated from decision making. Teachers who are informed about the issues of cochlear implantation are more likely to have dialogues with parents considering implants for their children and assume a role in candidacy selection.

With the intent of providing an organized listing of all factors considered for candidacy by one implant center, the Children's Implant Profile (ChIP), developed by the staff at Manhattan Eye, Ear & Throat Hospital (MEETH), is presented as an example of a decision-making tool.

■□ DEVELOPMENT OF THE ChIP

The early experiences of the cochlear implant center at MEETH provided information concerning children who had been successful or unsuccessful with their implant systems. A retrospective review of these cases generated data regarding certain factors that appeared with regularity in children who became successful users of the device. Borrowing the concept of the educational audiogram developed by Brookhauser and Moeller (1982), these factors were placed in a protocol that has become known as the Children's Implant Profile or ChIP.

The ChIP provides for a systematic evaluation of the child in a variety of areas that require input from each member of an interdisciplinary team. Each factor on the ChIP is operationally defined and graded according to the level of concern as noted by the team member responsible for that component. The levels of concern vary from no concern, mild to moderate concern, and great concern. When a factor is designated as being of mild to moderate or great concern, it implies that the potential benefit from the implant may be compromised as it relates to that factor. Thus, when complete, an individual profile of each child is available to use as both a counseling tool for the parents and as a decision-making device for the team (Hellman et al., 1991).

The 10 factors evaluated in the ChIP include the following: chronological age, duration of deafness, medical/radiological findings, multiple handicapping conditions, functional hearing ability, speech and language abilities, family structure and support, expectations of the family (parents and child), educational environment, and availability of support services (see Figure 4–1). The first four components of the ChIP are considered static in nature because they are physiologically based and are not amenable to direct remediation. In

CHILDREN'S IMPLANT PROFILE (ChIP)

NAME:
D.O.B.:   C.A.:
ETIOLOGY: ONSET: DURATION:
COMMUNICATION MODE:
SCHOOL PLACEMENT:

TEAM IMPRESSIONS OF THE FACTORS IMPORTANT TO IMPLANT USE AND SUCCESS	NO CONCERN	MILD-TO-MODERATE CONCERN	GREAT CONCERN
CHRONOLOGICAL AGE			
DURATION OF DEAFNESS			
MEDICAL/RADIOLOGICAL			
MULTIPLE HANDICAP			
FUNCTIONAL HEARING			
SPEECH & LANGUAGE ABILITIES			
FAMILY STRUCTURE & SUPPORT			
EXPECTATIONS			
EDUCATIONAL ENVIRONMENT			
AVAILABILITY OF SUPPORT SERVICE			

Figure 4–1
Children's Implant Profile (ChIP). (From Hellman et al. [1991]. The development of a children's implant profile. *American Annals of the Deaf, 136,* 77–81. Used with permission.)

contrast, the latter 6 factors can be controlled to a certain extent by professional intervention. Functional ability or status in each of the areas on the ChIP is determined by the team according to the definitions which follow.

Chronological Age

The *chronological age* component accounts for the child's age at the time of candidacy evaluation. If a child is between the ages of 4 and 10 years, there is no concern. Children of this age group are generally mature enough to actively participate in the testing procedure.

Children who are 2 and 3 years of age are considered to be of mild to moderate concern because oftentimes their ability to perform certain tasks is limited. These limitations may be developmental in nature; however, they are not inherent to the hearing-impaired population. Attention to task is necessary for evaluation and postimplant programming. A child must demonstrate a minimally acceptable level of attention and compliance in order to proceed with candidacy evaluation. A clear stimulus-response paradigm must be in the child's repertoire; if it is not present, training is necessary to establish this behavior.

Children between the ages of 11 and 18 are classified as causing great concern. Prior experience with preadolescent and adolescent children has shown a large number of nonusers and poor performers in this group (Chute, 1993). The problems of adolescence may be exacerbated in some individuals when an implant is recommended. Not only are cosmetic issues of concern but also issues of self-image and identity must be considered (Evans, 1989). More often than not, well-intentioned parents bring the teenager to the evaluation process with little or no explanation as to the nature of the visit. Additionally, teenagers themselves may be unrealistic about their performance with the device in the area of speech production. For this population, major improvements in speech intelligibility are unlikely. Unless this issue is addressed at the time of the evaluation, teenagers will be disappointed and may reject the device. For teenagers, the importance of preimplant counseling and training cannot be overstated. Networking potential candidates with implant recipients matched for age, duration of deafness, and communication style has proven to be useful in educating the adolescent candidate. Additionally, school counseling should be in place to provide support throughout the process. (See Chapter 10 for a complete discussion of rehabilitation strategies for teenagers.)

Duration of Deafness

The length of time that the child has sustained a bilateral sensorineural hearing loss is assessed under the factor *duration of deafness*. This issue addresses the plasticity of the auditory system as well as the period of deprivation as it relates to its resiliency. There is no concern if the duration of deafness is less than 4 years. Children who present with chronological ages of 2–3 years will automatically fall into this category. Often, children who have had meningitis at older ages will also likely present with short durations of deafness. Now that the cochlear implant is readily available, parents of children who contract meningitis will often seek an implant as soon as the youths are physically well.

Mild to moderate concern is noted if the duration of deafness is greater than 4 years but less than 8 years. This may include children who are congenitally deaf or early deafened and who have not sought an implant until they are older. A number of postmeningitic children can also be found in this category. As the duration of deafness increases, the degree of benefit from the device becomes less predictable. Because of the limited availability of the device during the period of investigation, parents may not have had the opportunity to apply for candidacy at that time due to geographical or financial constraints.

Finally, for children whose duration of deafness is greater than 8 years, there is great concern. This category includes those teenagers who were pre- or perilinguistically deaf. Here issues of auditory plasticity might negatively impact on the degree of benefit and the expediency with which the gains from the device can be observed. Experience with cochlear implants has shown that as the duration of deafness increases, the benefits of the device decrease (Tyler, 1993).

Medical/Radiological Results

Medical/radiological factors are assessed for each child being evaluated for a cochlear implant. The presence of congenital or acquired abnormalities of the cochlea or any other significant medical problem is determined. The etiology of the hearing loss, if known, is also carefully evaluated. Children whose hearing loss is secondary to meningitis often present with cochlear ossification. Ossification is abnormal bone growth on the cochlea that may restrict the number of electrodes that can be inserted into the inner ear. Malformed cochleas from congenital anomalies may also prevent the full insertion of all electrodes at the time of surgery (see Chapter 11 for performance results with this population). When the number of electrodes is severely limited, the performance of the child receiving the implant may be reduced (Parisier & Chute, 1993).

There is no concern if the cochleas are normal and unoccluded by any bony growth. This will allow the surgeon to easily insert the entire electrode array. Mild to moderate concern is recorded when the cochleas are partially ossified or not completely formed. In these cases, the surgeon may be able to introduce most, but not all, of the electrode array into the cochlea. Completely ossified cochleas or cochleas that are severely malformed create great concern and imply that certain special surgical steps be taken in order for the cochlea to receive the array. In these cases, the surgeon will only be able to insert 8–10 electrodes, thereby severely restricting the amount of information that can be transmitted.

Multiple Handicapping Conditions

The existence of any secondary handicap, either cognitive or physical in nature, is considered a *multiple handicapping condition*. Because signals from the cochlear implant are unlike normal hearing they may require more interpretation by the listener. If the child exhibits severe learning problems, the input may not be decipherable. Other handicapping conditions that may be related to motor coordination difficulties or those that are noncognitive in nature (e.g., blindness) are important to note, but will not likely impact the decision to implant (Chute & Nevins, 1995).

If the child exhibits no handicaps other than deafness, there is no concern by the evaluating team. There is mild to moderate concern for handicaps that are not cognitive but physical in nature (e.g., mild cerebral palsy). The reason for this mild concern is that rehabilitation strategies must be carefully planned to maximize input to the child and account for physical limitations. Great concern is noted when handicaps of a cognitive nature are involved because of the complexity of the implant signal. The Cochlear Implant Center at MEETH currently advises against implanting children who have severe secondary handicaps that fall into this category. Although there are some facilities that have implanted children with secondary cognitive handicaps (Bellman, 1994; Lesinski et al., 1994), these children have demonstrated limited success.

Functional Hearing Ability

The reliability of past audiological test results and the history of hearing aid use is assessed by the factor of *functional hearing ability*. Additionally, the ability of the child to perceive phonological contrasts when using either a hearing aid or a vibrotactile aid is evaluated as well. There is no concern if there is good reliability on audiological tests, a good history of hearing aid use, and evidence of auditory training. However, even though functional hearing ability is rated as being of no concern, a period of training with a tactile device may provide the audiologist with important information. Children who are unable to detect speech and make speech pattern contrasts through their hearing aids at the time of the initial evaluation may learn to discriminate these contrasts after tactile aid training. Thus, determining *true* functional hearing ability may require repeated evaluations, in addition to supervised preimplant training, in order to adequately exploit the child's response to auditory stimuli.

Assessment of hearing aid or vibrotactile aid benefit is one particular area in which the teacher can provide invaluable information to the evaluation team through the period of candidacy and preimplant training. Teachers instructing a child on a daily basis are capable of making observations over time to determine if the child has reached a plateau in speech and auditory abilities. This places the informed teacher in a position to offer information to the team regarding the child's auditory readiness for implantation.

Functional hearing ability is judged to be of mild to moderate concern when the reliability of the audiological testing is considered only fair and the history of hearing aid use and training is limited. Children presenting with this history must receive preimplant training directed by implant center personnel. Training will occur either through newly prescribed hearing aids or with a vibrotactile device. The decision to change amplification or prescribe a trial period with a vibrotactile aid is based on the results of the audiological testing performed at the center. When children with poor hearing aid histories are exposed to new amplification and/or vibrotactile stimulation they may learn to detect sound but do not learn to discriminate the patterns in speech. Many times these children are the younger of the implant candidates, which accounts for much of this behavior.

Children with good hearing aid histories may present with some pattern perception ability and even some word recognition. However, this is only accomplished under ideal listening conditions. Often, these children have been enrolled in aggressive auditory programs for a number of years and have reached a plateau in their auditory ability. Concern is rated as mild to moderate for these children because the process of implantation will destroy any residual hearing the child possesses at the time of candidacy.

Great concern is recorded for those children who have poor reliability in auditory testing situations and no history of hearing aid use or training. Before they can be evaluated effectively in this domain, these children need to be amplified appropriately and placed in a training program under the direction of the educational consultant from the implant team.

Auditory ability for children considered to be of great concern defines two distinct groups. The first group consists of those who possess too much residual hearing and do not exhibit commensurate auditory skills. This lack of auditory perceptual ability despite relatively good hearing aid responses may be indicative of an auditory processing problem. These children may not be able to effectively use the signal from the implant and should be considered poor candidates for implantation.

A second group of children who are considered to be of great concern for implantation are those who demonstrate no auditory reponses. These are often children who contracted meningitis and, subsequently, display a large degree of ossification (bone growth) on the cochlea. Stimulation from a cochlear implant may be compromised because of the bone growth limiting the amount of current which can be delivered, thereby restricting the benefits. For these children, the lack of response with hearing aids may leave them with very little choice. However, parents of these children need to be counseled carefully about the possibility of a reduced response.

Speech and Language Abilities

Assessing the *speech and language abilities* of children seeking cochlear implants is important to the decision-making process and the planning of a course for postoperative rehabilitation. While many implant centers perform language assessments solely as a baseline against which future performance will be measured, others view language competency as a critical component to implant success. From the perspective of the decision-making process, it is necessary to determine the sophistication of the child's linguistic system onto which new auditory percepts will be mapped. Given the child's age and duration of hearing loss, an underdeveloped language system may constrain the benefits derived from the implant. With regard to postoperative rehabilitation, speech-language evaluations provide a baseline from which to measure progress and identify the linguistic context in which to imbed auditory tasks. Language competence should be viewed as comprising both oral and manual modes of communication.

Additionally, it is meaningful to note the child's stimulability for speech. Although the majority of the children who are seen for cochlear implant evaluation have unintelligible speech, some measurement of their ability to approximate speech features should be performed. Because the cochlear implant is able to provide the deaf child with an enhanced auditory feedback system, and gains are expected in the area of speech intelligibility, obtaining a performance baseline is advised.

Speech and language abilities is yet another area in which local school professionals can be of great assistance. Personnel who have been monitoring the development of communication skills in a particular child are in a unique position to validate implant center findings. They may also be able to volunteer additional information with regard to a child's typical linguistic behavior. The classroom may provide a more natural setting in which the child's best linguistic performance may be demonstrated. This may be different from performance observed in a clinical, less familiar setting and is particularly common with young children. A cooperative effort between the implant center staff and local school personnel will ensure a truer assessment of the child's linguistic abilities.

There is no concern if a child's chronological age is equal to his linguistic age and he demonstrates that a formal language system is in place even if it is just developing. Mild to moderate concern is noted when there is a 1 to 3 year difference between the chronological age and language age. A formal language system may be in its emerging stages but there is good prognosis for development. There is great concern, however, if the difference between the language age and the chronological age is greater than 3 years or if no formal language system is demonstrated. As the gap between the chronological age and the linguistic age widens, there is serious question as to whether the child will be capable of interpreting the speech sounds he receives through the implant. These children will often be able to detect the presence of sound or the patterns of speech. However, there is little indication that the implant can provide the catalyst for language development that has failed to emerge using more traditional forms of instruction for the deaf.

Family Structure and Support

The involvement of the family in the overall rehabilitation process is assessed under the *family structure and support* component. Acceptance of the child's deafness is an important determinant in deciding cochlear implant candidacy. In addition, the ability of the family to augment the goals and objectives of the school program is also considered. The proficiency with which the parent communicates with the child (using whatever form of communication that has been chosen) is also important. Many parents demonstrate fluent and easy communication with their children using speech and/or sign language. Unfortunately, there are also families in which communication is labored and rudimentary at best. The structure of the family unit itself is also assessed. It is noted whether the child comes from a traditional family setting with both parents residing in the home or if the parents are divorced and/or remarried.

No concern is noted if the child comes from a traditional family setting and the family is able to communicate with the child using his preferred linguistic system. Parents who are actively involved with the child's language and academic program and provide him with opportunities to use his acquired skills at home also receive a no concern rating for this factor. There is mild to moderate concern when the child comes from a home environment in which the parents are divorced/remarried but both parents remain active in the child's life. It is helpful when stepparents are involved and able to cooperate in the (re)habilitative process as well. Great concern is evidenced when there is a single parent household with no input from the other parent in the care and management of the child. When the legal guardian of the child is neither the biological mother or father (other than in cases of adoption) great concern is also noted.

Expectations of the Family (Parents and Child)

Expectations of the family (parents and child) are evaluated regarding the projected benefit from a cochlear implant and whether they are realistic and appropriate. In the case of an adolescent candidate, expectations must be properly assessed. It is the practice at MEETH to counsel rather conservatively in order to minimize unrealistic expectations. The team acknowledges the existence of a range of performance ability after implantation. It is suggested that newfound auditory abilities may be limited to detection but not discrimination of speech. The ability to process patterns of speech and to recognize environmental sounds may be the extent of benefit for the device. Although many parents indicate they are interested solely in the "safety" factor, that is, having their child alert to a car horn, probing questions may reveal more lofty hopes.

There is no concern when the parent and child realize that the implant will not restore normal hearing and that the child will probably function in a manner similar to a child with a severe hearing loss. When parents expect that the implant will allow their child to move immediately from a self-contained classroom to a mainstream setting, there is mild to moderate concern. These parents may also believe that the need for educational support services will be eliminated. There is great concern when the parent or child anticipates that the implant will restore normal hearing. Clearly, these are counseling issues that must be resolved before a child can be implanted.

■□ EDUCATIONAL ENVIRONMENT

The appropriateness of the *educational environment* as it relates to the child's needs and abilities is carefully evaluated in the child's own school program. Children with implants have come from any one of a number of placement types: residential programs, regional day schools, day classes, resource rooms, and mainstream settings. The type of communication system used in the school is noted. Successful implant users may communicate using oral English, cued speech, or manually coded English with a simultaneous speech component. Regardless of placement type or communication methodology, the issue of school support for implantation is critical for maximizing benefit from the device.

When the school is supportive and able to provide flexible programming that matches the child's learning style and capabilities, there is no concern. School programs that have aggressive auditory management for all children are particularly appropriate for children with implants. Mild to moderate concern is noted when the school program is a good match with the child's capabilities but school personnel are uncertain about their own ability to provide proper management after the implant. These are programs in which teachers may not currently have the knowledge or skills necessary to manage a child postimplant but are willing to retool to address the child's needs. There is great concern when the school is found to be inflexible in its programming options, and it is not supportive of the use of sensory aids or auditory training. Children in this type of environment should not be considered candidates for a cochlear implant.

Availability of Support Services

Accessibility of the child/family to professionals in the areas of audiology, speech, language, and education of the hearing impaired is considered as part of the *availability of support services* factor. The degree and type of prior experience of the professionals relative to profoundly deaf children is also critical in evaluating this aspect of candidacy. The length of time devoted to follow-up habilitation is also assessed. MEETH recommends a *minimum* of three 30-minute sessions per week for speech and auditory activities.

There is no concern when there is access to experienced personnel on a daily basis. Mild to moderate concern is noted when access to personnel with limited experience is available once or twice a week. Although a speech and hearing professional need not have had direct experience with a child with an implant, familiarity with children with severe to profound hearing impairment is preferred. Finally, there is great concern when there is limited access to personnel with no special training in deafness. For children in rural areas, this rating is not uncommon as the low incidence of deafness impacts the availability of experienced personnel. When a school system has had difficulty in providing sufficient services on site, parents have supplemented therapy with outside professionals. In some cases, this has been supported by the school; however, in the majority of cases, parents have assumed this financial responsibility.

■□ CANDIDACY DECISION

Each child being considered a candidate for an implant is evaluated by the designated team member in each of the ChIP areas so that an individual profile is generated. This profile identifies the areas, if any, that must be remediated before a child can be considered for cochlear implant surgery. In all cases, the ChIP provides the team with a counseling tool so that performance projections based on a child's individual profile can assist the parents in making an informed decision should candidacy be recommended by the center. In general, three types of recommendations can be made by the implant center team after a final staffing of a candidate. First, implantation can be recommended because a majority of ChIP factors have been identified as being of no concern. Second, the decision to implant can be deferred until a later date because a number of ChIP items have been noted to be of mild to moderate or of great concern but are open to some intervention or remediation. A prime example of this type of decision is made for the young child who does not have the prerequisite skills to participate in postimplant tuning of the device. It is likely that with intensive training over time, the child will show readiness for the device, and candidacy would be reevaluated within a 6-month period.

Finally, there are selected cases in which implantation would not be recommended. These are cases for which a large number of ChIP items have been graded as being of great concern. An example of this type of case might be a child who exhibits secondary handicaps and whose performance with the device would be questionable.

◼◻ SUMMARY

The FDA has identified broad guidelines for candidate selection for pediatric cochlear implantation. These include profound deafness, showing little or no benefit from a hearing aid, and chronological age between 2 and 17 years. Many implant centers have identified additional criteria to help select children who may benefit from the potential of the device. The Children's Implant Profile enumerates 10 factors that are evaluated to determine implant candidacy. These include chronological age, duration of deafness, medical/radiological results, multiple handicapping conditions, functional hearing ability, speech and language abilities, family structure and support, expectations of the family (parents and child), educational environment, and availability of support services. Candidates are rated in each area on a scale of no concern, mild to moderate concern, and great concern. A profile is generated to assist the team in making its recommendation and to serve as a counseling tool for parents.

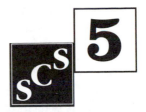

Supporting Parents Who Choose Implantation

The decision to seek implantation for a child is most often initiated by one or both of the child's parents. It is only in a few rare cases of adolescent implantation that the initial contact is made by the potential patient. The importance of parental and patient support is integral to the success of the process. A recommendation for a cochlear implant in a child may be made by a team; however, the final decision for implantation always rests with the parent (and the child). An informed consent that has been carefully explained and reviewed by the hearing health care professional is necessary before implant surgery can be performed. Exactly how a parent (and child) reaches that juncture will determine the future relationship between the family, the school and the cochlear implant team.

◼️ ESTABLISHING CONTACT

Parents most often contact the facility performing cochlear implants after speaking with other parents whose children have already received the device. In many cases, the children with implants are in the same class or school as the children whose parents are considering the surgery. Parents of unimplanted children often remark that, having observed the changes that took place in children after they received the cochlear implant, they made the decision to seek information for their own child. It is not unusual to have groups of children with implants centered within the same class or school. This grouping of children has been termed the "cluster phenomenon" (Chute, 1992) and represents a considerable amount of the pediatric cochlear implant population today.

On the surface, the information highway that has developed among parents at schools seems very efficient in disseminating first level knowledge to the families about the device. However, there is always a danger when parents make comparisons between the performance of one child with another. It becomes the responsibility of the implant team to dissuade well-meaning mothers and fathers from making these associations. An intensive and realistic appraisal of a child is necessary so that parents can understand the child's individual strengths, weaknesses, and potential to benefit from the device. How these strengths and weaknesses contribute to overall performance will assist the parents in deciding whether the cochlear implant is best for their child.

There are four stages of implantation through which parents (and their children) will require support. Successfully negotiating the evaluation, surgical, primary, and long-term rehabilitation stages necessitates a cooperative effort among the professionals at the implant facility, the teachers at the school, the parents of other implanted children, and the members of the family considering the implant. The role which each of these individuals plays in the support process will be important to the overall success of the child who receives the cochlear implant.

■❑ THE EVALUATION STAGE

Support Between the Cochlear Implant Center and the Family

Cochlear implant facilities should provide support for parents from the time of the first communication with that center. Although basic information about the cochlear implant is available from the manufacturers, it is most often disseminated through the implant facility.

Occasionally, parents obtain this information by contacting the manufacturer directly via hotlines or by attending conventions or forums. Nonetheless, once a parent has approached a particular center about an implant, it is the responsibility of the center to provide the parent with as much information as possible. As a result of the initial contact, the parent should receive written materials about the implant itself, the services which the center will supply, the estimated costs, and the names of other families who have already been through the process. These should be families who have indicated their willingness to speak with prospective parents and who have children with similar ages and durations of deafness.

Once a family contacts a center, both parents should be encouraged to attend the initial appointment, as long as the family structure allows for it. If multiple visits are warranted for evaluation purposes, it is not necessary for both parents to be available for every visit. However, at least one appointment during the process should include the mother and the father. For family situations in which there is a divorce and remarriage, it is recommended that the new extended family members be involved as well. For single-parent households, any additional caretakers for the child (e.g., grandparents, aunts, uncles, babysitters) should also receive information and be counseled.

The parents or legal guardians should be kept informed of the child's progress through the evaluation process. Concerns about the child should be carefully outlined. Counseling is performed best when using an objective tool such as the Children's Implant Profile (ChIP) (see Chapter 4). This profile allows the clinician a precise method of addressing each area of evaluation and how that area might affect the child's performance with the implant.

Parents should have an opportunity to see and handle the cochlear implant equipment. This should include both the internal receiver and the external hardware. Issues regarding postoperative restrictions and the possibility of an internal receiver failure should also be addressed. Financial aspects of implants should be reviewed at this time. Often, parents are concerned as to whether insurance companies pay for the device and what their financial obligations will be. They must be advised of the cost of follow-up visits postoperatively and the recurring costs associated with equipment upgrades. Many parents have already experienced this phenomenon as children have progressed from using the Nucleus WSP III to the MSP and now the Spectra. Although most insurance companies are willing to pay for the surgery and the initial cost of the device, there is no clearcut policy regarding the handling of expenses after initial implantation. Parents must be informed that there may be charges involved after implant surgery which are not covered under their insurance plan.

Regardless of which aspect of the cochlear implant is being discussed, a well- informed parent is critical to the success of the process. Instilling a feeling of support through ongoing communication between the family and the cochlear implant facility provides a strong foundation for future cooperation. If the implant staff creates an atmosphere of trust, parents will feel free to ask questions they may otherwise be afraid to voice.

Support Between the Cochlear Implant Center and the School

Because the school is the location to which the child will return (and on many occasions, the last to learn of the child's impending implant), it is imperative to include school personnel in the evaluation process. Immediate contact with the school will assist the implant team in assessing the whole child. Although direct contact by the cochlear implant facility is essential, parents must also take responsibility for informing the school about their decision to seek an implant for their child. Materials similar to those distributed to the parents should be made available to the school system as well. On-site evaluation of the child in the classroom, with input from the classroom teacher, will foster a cooperative relationship which can continue after implantation. The educational consultant model (see Chapter 2) best serves these purposes.

Although it is the educational consultant who is designated to act as the liaison between the implant facility and the school, in reality, it is the parent who must maintain daily contact to ensure that the educational plan is being followed. Some parents come to the implant process with a history of interacting with their child's school; others do not have much experience in this area. Encouraging the parents to become integral members of their child's educational team should begin at the time of the initial contact. An important function of the educational consultant is in empowering the parents to assume the lead role in communicating with the teaching and therapeutic staff.

Support Between the Family and the School

Parents with children who are congenitally deaf are usually, but not always, more knowledgeable about the special educational process because they have spent more time within the system. Parents of children who are newly diagnosed or have acquired deafness have little knowledge about their child's educational needs. These parents often do not know the proper questions to raise in negotiating for special education services. Issues regarding the degree and type of therapy the child should be receiving, who should be dispensing these services, and whether additional help is necessary must be addressed.

Many times parents begin seeking an implant for their child without ever informing the school of their intent, thereby precluding input from the individuals who know the child well. Parents report that they are fearful of informing the school about their child's implant candidacy because the educational personnel may have preconceived notions which are not supportive of this technology. This results in the parents feeling alienated by the school when the evaluation process is begun. The situation becomes exacerbated if the implant center excludes the school during the early phases of implantation and wreaks havoc later during the (re)habilitation stage. Encouraging the parents to inform the school of their interest in the implant will help to build a cooperative relationship that can only be positive.

Support From Other Parents
of Implanted Children

One of the most important contacts that parents make is with other families of children with implants. Occasionally, families who are seeking implants have already met other families of implanted children. However, even if this is the case, every attempt should be made to place the parents of the implant candidate in contact with a family who has already been through the process. Since the evaluation phase is often filled with anxiety and doubt, communicating with other families and learning about their experiences is often helpful. Facilitating that introduction is a key role which the implant center plays.

■☐ THE SURGICAL STAGE

Support Between the Family
and the Implant Center

Issues regarding surgery and the logistics of the hospital stay should be carefully reviewed with the family by implant personnel.

Oftentimes, parents are unaware of the hospital regulations regarding entrance into the surgical suite or overnight visitation with the child. Many hospitals do not permit parents to enter the surgical suite; it is recommended that a member of the team, who is well known to the child, accompany him. Parents should be reminded that the child will have a large bandage on his head after the surgery; therefore, pajamas and clothing for the trip home should be the type that button down the front. For older children, provisions should be made for assistive devices and closed caption television. Postoperatively, information about bathing, physical activities, and return appointments also need to be addressed. Because this period is often a stressful one, it is best to provide this information to the parent in both spoken and written form (see Appendix B).

After the surgery, a visit to the family by an implant team member fosters continued feelings of support and decreases feelings of abandonment. This visit provides the parents with an opportunity to ask questions and creates a bridge into the next phase of the process.

Support Between the Implant Center and the School

It is not unusual to all but forget the school during the surgical stage because it is not directly involved in this portion of the implantation process. This lack of involvement on the part of the school should not be confused with lack of concern. Many times, the classroom teacher and therapists, who have been an integral part of the child's life, are as concerned about the surgical procedure as the parents themselves. With permission from the parents, a report to the school about the surgery should be sent as soon as possible. Telephone contact on the day of the surgery is often appreciated. Communication with the school about the surgery should include information regarding the number of electrodes implanted, the projected date of initial device setting, and postoperative restrictions. Often the school is concerned about any limitations of physical activities (e.g., in the playground or in physical education classes) during the immediate recuperative period.

Support Between the Family and the School

The family should be encouraged to communicate with the school during the surgical period. Immediate communication regarding the outcome of the surgery should be part of the parental responsibility to the educational setting. Although additional information should be provided by the implant center, the family's personal knowledge of the teacher and therapists involved with their child will help to maintain the family/school connection.

Support From Parents of Implanted Children

Parents often find it helpful to discuss the fears and apprehensions of surgery with other parents who have already been through the process. Because all parents should have made contact with at least one family whose child has already received an implant, the support for this phase often comes from the same family. In many cases, families begin a long-lasting relationship with other families who they have met during the initial stages of implantation.

■□ REHABILITATION STAGE

Support Between the Implant Center and the Family

The rehabilitation stage is the longest and most critical of all the phases of cochlear implantation. This period can be divided into a primary and a long-term stage. The primary phase of rehabilitation, which encompasses the tune-up and therapy immediately following it, is the most stressful for parents. It is at this time that parental expectations are high and knowledge level regarding outcomes is low. Even for sophisticated parents who have a large information base regarding hearing aid acoustics, auditory perception, and linguistic competence, the technology of electrical stimulation and "tuning" the implant is likely to be foreign. Some centers find it helpful to provide parents with a dictionary of implant terms (see Appendix C for a dictionary of terms for Nucleus device and Appendix D for a dictionary of terms for the Clarion device) that are used during the tune-up session. For parents with less sophistication, the concepts of electrodes and current and their relationship to hearing with the implant may be extremely difficult to comprehend. Written materials which are available prior to the tune-up provide each parent with the opportunity to be exposed to the new language and vocabulary of cochlear implants so that they might understand more of the device-tuning process. Written materials, however, should never be a replacement for face-to-face explanations. Additionally, correspondence about the amount and type of external equipment which will be distributed, the time commitment involved, and the costs for the initial tune-up should be sent to parents soon after surgery (see Appendix E).

Whenever possible, a soundfield audiogram should be performed after the initial tune-up. Although thresholds from this audiogram may be slightly elevated, it provides the clinician with a mechanism to discuss the initial auditory capabilities of the child using legends and techniques that are more familiar to the parents. Since most parents are familiar with reading an audiogram, much of the tune-up procedure can be demystified by relating it to this more accustomed form. Information regarding the initial responses which were observed while the child first wore the device should be reviewed with the parents so that therapeutic objectives appropriate for that level of performance can be developed (see Chapter 6). Setting realistic goals for the child so that the parents are not disappointed is critical at this juncture of the implant process. Strategies for providing auditory input and encouraging speech output should be presented in a clear and understandable manner.

Oftentimes, with very young implant recipients (e.g., 2-year-old children), parents must initially spend a great deal of time in reinforcing the child's acceptance of the device. To avoid frustration and feelings of inadequacy, it is crucial for the implant center to provide support for parents should wearing issues occur during these early stages (see Chapter 8). Ongoing communication via telephone calls should aid the parents through this period.

After the initial stimulation, and before leaving the implant facility, parents must be trained in the wear and care of the device as well as troubleshooting techniques. This process is made easier if an actual demonstration of the strategies is performed. To ensure proper carryover in the home, written and sometimes videotape materials should be distributed (see Appendix F which outlines procedures for the Nucleus device and Appendix G which outlines procedures for the Clarion device).

The primary stage of rehabilitation often sets the tone for future communication with the parents. If support is weak or nonexistent at this phase of implantation, the likelihood of its improving over time is slim. Because the cochlear implant facility represents that segment of the support system with the most knowledge about the device, it is imperative that the clinical team involved with the child be available for any and all questions.

The emphasis during the long-term stage of rehabilitation shifts from the concerns and notions involved with the tune-up to the overall progress that the child is making with the device. This stage is under the care of a variety of team members. The audiologist should deal with those issues directly related to the functioning of the device and the appropriateness of the emerging auditory abilities. Discussions with the parents should include information about the need to retune the device periodically and the schedule for when this might occur. Equipment problems or concerns should also be addressed. Strategies which the parents are using to foster good listening and speaking behavior should be reviewed. Direct input regarding the speech skill development and speech targets that should be emphasized can be discussed by the speech-language pathologist. Approaches used to develop vocabulary and linguistic competence that is age appropriate for the child should also be presented at this time.

The educational consultant should be available to discuss with the parents the carryover of behaviors from the classroom. Fostering a good relationship postoperatively with the school and the family is key to good long-term follow-up. Information discussed with the school regarding the child's performance in the classroom can be reinforced by the educational consultant when meeting with the parents.

Finally, communication with the surgeon who performed the implant should not cease. Parents should be certain to inform the otologist of any ear infections or serious illnesses that the child may have sustained since his last evaluation. Although parents can continue to seek their pediatrician's intervention for treatment of childhood illnesses, they should make certain that correspondences regarding these visits are forwarded to the implant surgeon.

Good follow-up by the center after implantation will provide parents with information about any technological advances in a timely fashion. Proper communication with the implant facility will provide the link between the manufacturer and the patient necessary to provide the best service possible for the implant recipient.

Support Between the Center and the School

The educational consultant model requires ongoing communication between the implant facility and the educational setting. This is important during all phases of rehabilitation. At the primary stage, school personnel need to become knowledgeable about the many aspects of implantation. This information is best transmitted through an on-site visit by the educational consultant. At that time, an explanation of the tune-up, the performance of the child on the first day of stimulation, and initial therapeutic strategies are reviewed. Troubleshooting techniques and maintenance information about the device are areas in which the school personnel should be knowledgeable. The school personnel should feel as if they are an integral part of the rehabilitative process for the child. If they have been ignored during the prior stages, there may be feelings of hostility, making the rehabilitation phase less productive. Fostering good communication between the center and the school helps support the parents of the implanted child.

The second portion of the rehabilitation phase encompasses the long-term follow up. The ongoing therapy for the implant recipient is most often delivered in the educational setting. Although there may be instances in which children have additional therapy provided privately, the majority of the direct services will be supplied here. Since habilitative needs will change over time both within the same school year as well as between years (Nevins, 1994), it is important that information regarding auditory and speech progress be conveyed to the educational setting. Subsequent site visits by the educational consultant may become necessary for children who are experiencing difficulties in the classroom. Changes in the support systems available for the child may also become an issue. This problem may be addressed more appropriately through the educational liaison who is knowledgeable about cochlear implants and the education of hearing-impaired children. Educational intervention by an implant center educator supports parents who have neither the knowledge nor the skill to negotiate the system on their child's behalf.

Support Between the Family and the School

The initial stages of cochlear implant rehabilitation are fraught with anxiety and uncertainty. This uncertainty on the part of the parent is eased through the support of the implant facility. The school's uncertainty can be assuaged by the educational consultant. However, it is important for the parent and the school to forge a good working relationship, because their partnership will be ongoing. Parents should make certain that teachers and therapists involved with their child voice any concerns or questions at this primary stage of rehabilitation. Likewise, the school should expect numerous inquiries from the parents seeking information about the child's progress during this initial phase. Many parents need a great deal of positive reinforcement at this period in the rehabilitation. This reinforcement will come from teachers who may be able to discriminate small changes in the child's auditory behavior. Additionally, it might be teacher input that alerts the parent to a need for remapping. (Remapping is required periodically as the child's perception of sound changes. These changes are electronically written onto the memory of the speech processor.) Constant dialogue between the family of the implanted child and the school ensures a good working association which benefits the child.

As the duration of implant use increases, the needs of the child in the classroom will also change. As the academics become more challenging, both the teacher and the parent may find it necessary to alter programs which have been successful up to this point. If teacher/parent interaction has been consistent, these changes can occur with ease and cooperation. If there has been little communication between the family and the school, feelings of conflict may result. Acting as the intermediary for parents who have not had good communication with the school, the implant facility's educational consultant may work to improve the home/school link. This will make the long-term goals for the rehabilitation of the child with the cochlear implant truly a cooperative effort.

Support From Parents of Implanted Children

Parents who have already experienced the initial tune-up of their child with a cochlear implant are often some of the best resources for parents who are facing the process. The range of emotion on the first day of stimulation can vary from elation to disappointment. Most parents experience a feeling between these two. It is helpful, especially for parents whose children may not have performed as well on the first day, to speak with other parents who may have had similar experiences. For other parents whose children may have performed very well initially, anxiety may surface later when the child reaches a plateau in performance. Finally, there are times when the internal receiver may cease to function and another surgery becomes necessary. Parents (and children) who have had similar experiences are an extremely important resource at this very trying time. For most parents of children with cochlear implants, there is a tremendous feeling of gratitude which is evidenced when these same parents demonstrate their willingness to act as a resource to new families as they begin the process of implantation.

◼◻ RESOURCES FOR PARENTS

The importance of parent-to-parent (and patient-to-patient) contact is paramount to the success of cochlear implant evaluation and rehabilitation. Many states have separate cochlear implant clubs or meet in conjunction with the local chapter of the A.G. Bell Association. Cochlear Implant Club International (CICI) has existed since the early days of cochlear implantation and sponsors yearly conferences. These meetings serve as a forum in which people can meet and learn about advances and practicalities in the field of cochlear implants. All cochlear implant recipients should be encouraged to become members in both the local and national organizations.

◼◻ SUMMARY

Supporting parents who seek cochlear implants for their children is a primary responsibility for centers with a pediatric program. Clinicians involved in implantation have found that a large portion of their clinical time is spent in speaking with families, alleviating their anxieties, and providing emotional support as their children progress through the various stages of cochlear implant use. Although a great deal of the responsibility for training the child rests with the school, the parent must maintain an active role in this process. The parent is the connecting link between the child's educational facility and the implant facility. Cooperation and support must come from the implant facility, school, and other parents who have already been through the process. With the assistance of the implant center, parents must be guided in exploiting all the resources available to them.

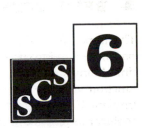

Designing a Management Program for Children with Implants

Proper management of the child after implantation is a cooperative effort among the team members at the cochlear implant center, the school, and the parents. The initiating activity of the postimplant phase is the tune-up of the external speech processor. This event occurs approximately 4–6 weeks after the surgery. With rare exception, an initial tune-up session lasts for 2 days. During that time, the device is turned on and set according to the child's needs. Parents (and any other professionals or family members who are present) are trained in the maintenance and troubleshooting aspects of the unit. Contraindications regarding medical treatment are also reviewed.

■□ THE INITIAL TUNE-UP

Generally, for children below the age of 7, two audiologists are required to perform the tune-up procedure. Standard pediatric audiological testing techniques which incorporate traditional reinforcement paradigms are used. The test procedure requires the child to respond to an electrical signal that is delivered to each electrode individually. Testing begins with the low frequency electrodes, typically electrode 20 in the Nucleus device. (The newest device, the Clarion, is numbered so that the low frequency electrodes begin with electrode 1.) The specific procedure described herein is for the Nucleus implant. Tune-up techniques are similar among all implants; however, certain nuances related to the particular design of each implant may require a departure from the general procedures outlined below.

Although some audiologists program children in a stimulation mode known as common ground (CG), the majority of children are now programmed in bipolar plus one (BP+1) stimulation mode. To understand these terms and exactly what the tune-up accomplishes, it is necessary to appreciate the dynamics of delivering electrical current to a system. Electricity must always flow between two points. An active electrode is one half of the electrode pair which begins the stimulation. The indifferent electrode is the other half of the pair which acts as the ground for the current. Depending on the proximity of the electrodes to one another, the flow of current can be extremely wide or very narrow. When the active and indifferent electrode are next to one another, it is known as bipolar (BP) stimulation. If there is one electrode between the active and the indifferent, it is known as bipolar plus one (BP+1). As the number of electrodes between the active and the indifferent increases, the spread of current will widen. These stimulation modes are termed BP+2, BP+3, and so on. When a common ground mode (CG) is used, one electrode is chosen as the active. All the remaining electrodes are connected together and become the indifferent (Cochlear Corporation, 1994). The mode of electrical stimulation is important because it determines how much current is necessary for the child to respond. There may be occasions in which there are limitations on the amount of current that can be delivered to the implant recipient.

Multichannel electrode arrays utilize multiple electrodes placed in the cochlea in a predetermined manner. These electrodes are assigned certain frequency bands. The low frequency bands are located toward the apical end of the cochlea, and the high frequency bands are located at the basal end. The location of the bands with regard to frequency response has been designed in an attempt to mimic the frequency allocation which is exhibited in the normal cochlea.

The tune-up procedure requires that the child's speech processor be connected to an interface box which communicates with a computer. The headset (which includes the microphone and the transmitter coil) is placed on the child's head over the area of the internal receiver (see Figure 6–1). Because profoundly deaf children often have a better percept of low frequency sound, it is customary that a low frequency electrode be stimulated first. The initial task is to determine the threshold level for a particular electrode. Electrical pulses are delivered to a designated electrode at a particular current level determined by the audiologist using a control knob. This control knob regulates the delivery of the pulses and is graded numerically from units of 1 through 239. These units are arbitrary and do not equate to decibel levels.

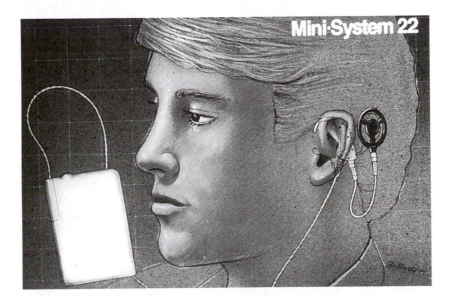

Figure 6–1
Headset in place. (Photograph courtesy of Cochlear Corporation.)

Assessing Threshold and Comfort Levels

The control knob is turned gradually until the child either acknowledges hearing a sound or, behaviorally, is observed to have heard a sound. Often, in the young child, this may be an orienting response or a head turn. In older children, standard play audiometry techniques and/or behavioral observation methods are used to obtain responses. The lowest level at which the child consistently identifies sound sensation is designated as the threshold or T-level. T-levels are obtained for each of the active electrodes.

In addition to obtaining T-levels for each electrode, another electrical response is also measured. This electrical value is determined by continuing to increase the amount of current being delivered to the electrode (via the control knob) until the child reports a comfortably loud sensation. This measurement is known as the comfort level or C-level. With the Clarion device, these levels are referred to as the M-level (see Appendix D). Since many children do not have a well developed concept of sound, assessing comfort may be too abstract a task, making C-levels difficult to obtain. Of utmost importance is the audiologist's ensuring that the signal delivered to the electrode is not *un*comfortable.

In an attempt to obtain an objective measure of the C-level in children, research has been conducted using the electrically elicited stapedial reflex (EART) (Hodges, Ruth, Thomas, & Blincoe, 1991; Spivak & Chute, 1994). The EART (**E**lectro**A**coustic **R**eflex **T**hreshold) is a measurement made using standard tympanometric recordings. This procedure requires that a rubber tip be placed in the ear canal to seal off any air. The air pressure in the canal is manipulated in order to record information about the movement of the eardrum. Simultaneously, a sound is delivered to the opposite ear. When sound reaches a particular level in the opposite ear, a tiny muscle in the middle ear will contract and move the eardrum. This contraction is known as the acoustic reflex and protects the normal hearing ear from loud sounds. Eardrum movement as a result of the acoustic reflex can be measured in implanted children and adults by stimulating the cochlear implant in one ear and recording the reflex in the opposite ear. These measurements have been successfully used to provide clinicians with a more objective assessment of C-levels.

When comfort levels are extremely high (i.e., over 200 units) there may be a need to change to a different stimulation mode. If a child is being programmed in BP+1 and exhibits very high C-levels, switching to a different stimulation mode (e.g., BP+2) will spread the current across a wider area. This functionally decreases the amount of current necessary to reach the C-level. For children who have had meningitis and exhibit bone growth on their cochlea, more current may be required to stimulate the neural tissue. For this reason, BP+1 may not be an efficient method of delivering the signal, because the available current will produce a sound that has a reduced growth of loudness. Exploration of other stimulation modes by the programming audiologist will allow for the best possible program for the child.

Creating the Map

When threshold (T-levels) and comfort (C-levels) have been obtained for each of the electrodes, a program is developed using the manufacturer's software. This program, in the Nucleus device, is known as a *map* and is somewhat similar to the frequency specifications of a conventional hearing aid (Myres & Kessler, 1992). However, it is much more specific to the individual patient. For the Clarion device, it is simply referred to as a *program*. A sample map can be found in Figure 6–2 for the Nucleus device. The Clarion device program is shown in Figure 6–3.

The map contains information about the threshold and comfort levels and the frequency boundaries for each of the programmed electrodes. These frequency boundaries have a particular relationship with respect to the number of electrodes assigned to them. A designated number of electrodes are allocated to frequencies above and below 1000 Hz. Clinicians programming children in the traditional MPEAK strategy with the Nucleus device (see Chapter 3) may restrict the number of electrodes initially placed in the map. This decision is often made when children exhibit a sensitivity to the presence of high frequency sounds. Although there are occasions when the high frequency *electrodes* might have been left out of the map, it should be understood that high frequency *information* is still being delivered to the child. In those cases in which the quantity of electrodes has been restricted, the range of band frequencies mapped to each electrode is greater. When electrodes are restricted, the tolerance for high frequency sound improves. Regardless, limiting electrode number is usually a condition of early implant mapping and as the child adapts to the signal, electrodes are added over time. High frequency definition is inconsequential at this stage of implant use, because the child is first acclimating to the presence of sound as opposed to the finer nuances of speech stimuli.

Fri May 26 09:49:59 1995

Summary of map 7 created on 26-May-95 at 09:37 with V6.90
The T stimulus level has been modified by 0%
The C stimulus level has been modified by 0%
Mode = BP+1 Base Level = 4 Encoder Strategy: SPEAK
Optimum Sensitivity Setting = 3.0 for Spectra 22 338499
Loudness Growth Q value = 20 Autosensitivity on S Position = Yes
Number of maxima = 6
Frequency allocation Table = 7

Elect.	T-level	C-level	Range	Freq. Bounds Lower	Upper	Gain
20	95	189	94	120	280	8
19	92	188	96	280	440	8
18	91	185	94	440	600	8
17	76	170	94	600	760	8
16	91	183	92	760	920	8
15	88	180	92	920	1080	8
14	94	185	91	1080	1240	8
13	80	170	90	1240	1414	8
12	97	194	97	1414	1624	8
11	100	189	89	1624	1866	8
10	109	197	88	1866	2144	8
9	83	183	100	2144	2463	8
8	67	170	103	2463	2856	8
7	87	177	90	2856	3347	8
6	66	160	94	3347	3922	8
5	96	195	99	3922	4595	8
4	84	188	104	4595	5384	8
3	78	180	102	5384	6308	8
2	83	183	100	6308	7390	8
1	63	170	107	7390	8658	8

Figure 6–2
Sample Map for the Nucleus 22 Channel Cochlear Implant.

Mapping strategies have changed somewhat with the introduction of the new generation of the Nucleus device. The Spectra 22 incorporates a strategy known as SPEAK (see Chapter 3) which does not appear to present the same difficulties with respect to the acceptance of high frequency information by children. For this reason, children initially tuned with the Spectra will probably utilize all active electrodes.

The Clarion device has a unique feature; the speech processor is capable of storing multiple programs. This option enables the audiol-

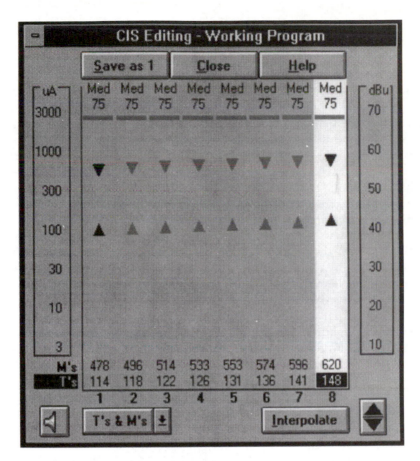

Figure 6–3
Sample Program for the Clarion Multi-Strategy Cochlear Implant.

ogist to set the device in three different ways. Often, the initial setting will reflect the T-levels and M-levels obtained during the tune-up session. The second program might also utilize the T- and M-levels obtained but emphasize or deemphasize high or low frequency information. A third program might emphasize the middle frequencies or increase intensity across all frequencies. The setting of these programs is left to the discretion of the audiologist. Therapists and parents need to be informed of the procedure for selecting new programs and the content of each. The practical application of the Clarion's capability of storing additional programs is that the child and the parent or teacher can work interactively to select the most appropriate setting.

Once a speech processor has been programmed with a particular map for a particular child, **no other child should use that child's speech processor**. Using another child's processor can present signals which are painful and may create a negative attitude toward the device. Periodically, as a child's auditory perceptual performance changes, his map may also need adjustment. This requires the child to return to the implant facility so that new T and C levels can be obtained and a new program can be written to the microchip of the speech processor. Most implant centers request that children return for frequent follow-up visits for the first 6 months of implant use. As the child's responses with the implant stabilize, the need for additional mapping sessions tends to decrease.

In many cases, the linguistic constraints of very young children, coupled with their lack of auditory experience, prevent them from indicating when a remapping is necessary. In these instances, observations by the parents and the school teachers are invaluable in signaling when a mapping change is warranted. There are certain signs indicative of a need for remapping which teachers and parents should recognize. Children who suddenly begin to increase the sensitivity of their device from the baseline setting (see the following section on Function and Sensitivity Controls) may discover that the perceived increase in loudness which results from this change allows them to hear better. This is usually a sure sign that the child is in need of more power from the speech processing unit. Generally, when these children are remapped, clinicians find that there have been large increases in comfort levels.

Additionally, changes in speech production may be a signal that the child's speech processor needs to be remapped. Sudden changes in vocalizations or loss of speech features that the child was previously able to produce may be an indication that a remapping is necessary. Finally, if the child suddenly develops a physical symptom, (e.g., an eye or facial twitch or sensation in the neck or tongue), an appointment with the implant center should be made immediately. Physical manifestations or unusual sensations may require the deletion of electrodes which are causing problems.

It is extremely important that the implant facility, the parent, and the school maintain good communication to determine the child's need for a remapping. Contact with the cochlear implant facility will enable the relationship between the center and the school to continue in a cooperative manner.

■ THE NUCLEUS DEVICE: DESCRIPTION OF CONTROLS

Function and Sensitivity Controls

There are two control dials on the speech processor available for adjustment by the parent, teacher, or child. The first of these is the function switch which controls the input to the processor. For the Nucleus device, there are four positions. The "N" position is the traditional setting used to activate the unit. The "O" position turns the unit off. The "T" setting is used to test the battery life. The "S" position is a noise suppression setting (see Figure 6–4). Appropriate device settings for the child are reviewed with the parents at the time of the initial tune-up. Although little deviation should occur from these settings, it is important to understand how changes in the prescribed control dial positions may affect the child's performance.

Most children, with rare exception, wear their speech processor on the "N" setting. If the classroom teacher notices that the child is not

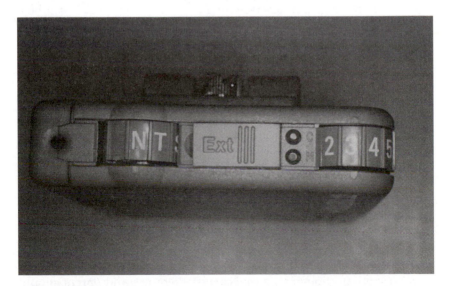

Figure 6–4
Function and sensitivity controls of the Nucleus 22 Channel Cochlear Implant.

as responsive as usual, she should check to make certain the unit is turned on. (A more detailed description of troubleshooting techniques is discussed later in this chapter.) There is a small group of children who use their processor in the "S" position; the implant center will determine the proper setting at the time of the tune-up and inform the parent and school about this decision. Under no circumstances should a child ever be wearing the unit in the "T" position. In fact, the headset should always be removed from the child when testing the batteries with this function setting. If the child is wearing the unit and the control dial is rotated into the "T" position, he may hear a continual high pitched sound which can be annoying or even uncomfortable. Should a teacher discover that a child is wearing the implant in the "T" position, it must be switched immediately to the "N" position and the parents informed.

The second control located on the top of the Nucleus speech processor adjusts the sensitivity of the unit. This dial is numbered continuously from 1–8 and is often mistaken as a volume control. Although sensitivity settings will adjust the volume of the signal, to a certain degree, it should not be viewed as a traditional volume control. The sensitivity setting determines the responsiveness of the microphone. With a low sensitivity setting (e.g., 1–2), input to the microphone must be very close in proximity (i.e., speaker must be within a few inches of the microphone). With a high sensitivity setting (e.g., 7–8), the speaker can be a further distance away from the microphone (e.g., in a large lecture hall).

The sensitivity control is set via the computer during the tune-up process. Teachers and therapists should be informed (either by the parent or implant facility) of the appropriate setting for the child. Generally, sensitivity is set at level 3, 4, or 5. Often, when children are first adjusting to their implants, it is recommended that the parents initially set the unit at a very low sensitivity (e.g., 2). Over the course of the next few minutes, they should gradually increase it to the designated setting. Because deaf children have had limited exposure to sound, this precaution is taken to ensure they are not overstimulated when they first place their processors on each morning.

If, on the other hand, an increase in sensitivity becomes necessary for the child to maintain function, then the child may be due for a remapping of his speech processor. Until the parent is able to bring the child to the implant facility for a remapping, it is not harmful for the child to wear the processor at the higher sensitivity setting. Again, good communication among the teacher, therapist, and parent should help avoid long periods of the child's wearing the unit on a setting that is less efficient for him.

■□ THE CLARION DEVICE: DESCRIPTION OF CONTROLS

Function, Sensitivity, and Volume Control

The Clarion Multi Strategy Cochlear Implant System is designed with three separate control knobs for patient use (see Figure 6–5). The patient may select between different strategies or multiple programs of the same strategy by turning the Function mode switch on the speech processor. Other adjustable controls include the Volume and Sensitivity knobs. The Sensitivity knob behaves in a similar manner as described with the Nucleus device. Unlike the Nucleus device, there is also a separate Volume control knob to increase overall gain from the unit.

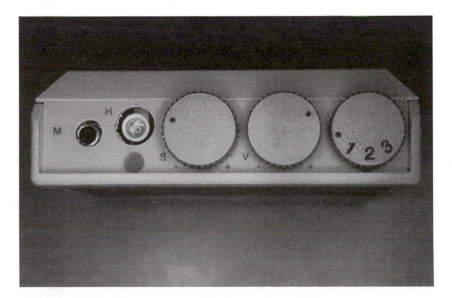

Figure 6–5
Device controls for the Clarion Multi-Surgery Implant.

◼□ RESPONSES OF CHILDREN AFTER THE INITIAL TUNE-UP

The range of performance which can occur after children have experienced their first stimulation with a cochlear implant can be divided into four groups. Group 1 encompasses the largest number of children who receive cochlear implants. This group of children is able to detect a wide range of speech signals (Ling 6 sounds as well as their own name). This detectability is exhibited only in structured tasks with specific listening paradigms (e.g., Put the block in the bucket when you hear the sound). The second group of children includes those implant users who are able to discriminate different patterns of speech after the initial tune up (e.g., cat vs. baseball). Again, this ability is only demonstrable in structured situations. The third group of children exhibits no auditory awareness of sound but wears the speech processor without any complaints or manifestation of aversive stimulation. This group often includes young children with limited communication skills; however, they have a positive attitude toward wearing the device. The fourth and last group encompasses those children who refuse to wear the device even when it is turned off. These children are often the very young who do not have the linguistic sophistication to understand or participate interactively in the tune-up process.

It is important that the therapeutic course developed for children with implants considers each child's response to initial stimulation. Table 6–1 outlines immediate postimplant auditory objectives based on this response. Many parents of children who refuse to wear the device must be taught behavioral modification techniques to assist them through this first stage (see Chapter 8). Other parents whose children show good detection and discrimination on the first day can begin the process of building their child's sound dictionary without delay.

The immediate goal for all children who receive cochlear implants is for detection of speech and environmental sounds. Parents should be trained in the process of providing listening opportunities in the home environment. Teachers likewise should provide similar listening experiences. Because detection of the child's name is an important step in this process, it provides a good starting point. Knowledge of one's name provides an individual with a reference point in both time and space. Once response to his name becomes automatic, a child becomes a more active participant in the world.

Detection of one's name, however, should not be the only goal at this immediate postimplant phase. Hearing and discriminating envi-

TABLE 6–1
Immediate Auditory Goals To Be Implemented Following the Initial Stimulation of the Device.

If the child:	Then initial teaching objective should encourage:
• detects a wide range of speech signals in structured tasks	• responding to name • perceiving pattern contrasts (single syllable words vs. multi-syllable words and/or short phrases or sentences vs. long phrases or sentences)
• discriminates different patterns of speech in structured situations (The largest percetage of children will begin at this level.)	• constant expansion of set of pattern contrasts • carryover of acquired skills demonstrated in structured setting to classroom • introduction to closed set listening tasks
• wears the processor but shows no auditory awareness	• alerting to the presence of speech sounds, especially the child's name • alerting to environmental sounds
• refuses to wear the device	• implementation of a wearing program • getting the device turned on as soon as possible and begin alerting to speech

ronmental sounds in the home and at school will offer the child the opportunity to begin to recognize the diversity of sound. If, after an extended program of aural habilitation, the child is unable to consistently detect sound in the environment, then success with the implant is questionable. The majority of children with cochlear implants eventually attain levels of performance which enable them to detect and discriminate among the various patterns of speech. Of this group, many will go beyond these skills and further develop the ability to recognize speech through listening alone (see Chapter 11). Although it is difficult to determine which children will develop this ability, proper auditory intervention is crucial to its growth.

■▢ CARE AND MAINTENANCE OF THE EXTERNAL EQUIPMENT

Teachers, parents, and when possible, the children themselves, should be taught the proper methods of maintaining the external portion of the cochlear implant system. If the device is carefully maintained on a daily or weekly basis, many simple problems that can arise can be avoided. Children's reliance on their cochlear implant warrants an appreciation for the method in which it functions and the necessity for proper upkeep. Many of the procedures used to maintain and care for cochlear implant equipment are similar to those used with traditional hearing aids. Although the burden of maintaining the unit rests on the child's parents (and/or the child), the teacher should also be aware of some of the issues of daily maintenance.

As with any electronic equipment, the first and foremost avoidable problem is related to physical abuse and moisture. Although most children wear their speech-processing units in some type of pouch or carrier, there are some locations of wear that are more subject to abuse. It is preferable, especially for the very young active child to situate the processor on the child's back in a protective pouch. This pouch is usually connected by means of a harness and is worn under his clothing. Effectively, this safeguards the unit in two ways. First, it removes the processor from the child's access thereby preventing him from changing the dial settings. Second, it protects the unit from exposure to damaging elements (e.g., water and food).

If the speech processor has been subject to physical abuse while at school, either intentional or accidental, the functioning of the device should be checked and the parents informed of the problem. Intentional abuse to the speech processor should be reported immediately to both the parents and the implant facility in order to determine the cause of the problem and resolve it. If a child is removing the unit in the classroom and deliberately throwing it, it may be behavior or map related. Map-related problems should be addressed by the implant center, whereas behavioral problems may require implementing behavior modification techniques at home and in school.

If, despite all the best intentions, the speech processor and/or headset has gotten wet while the child is at school, the teacher/therapist can provide some immediate care for the unit. First, the teacher should make certain that moisture has truly created a problem with the functioning of the unit. Determining processor function is easy if the child is able to articulate the breakdown. If the child is unable to tell the teacher that the processor sounds acceptable and the child's level of auditory perception is still at the rudimentary stage, then the unit should be turned off and the parents should be informed. No attempt should be made by the teacher to dry out the unit. Parents have been trained in the procedures to be used when this occurs. (See Appendix F or G for a complete description of these techniques.)

In much the same way that moisture can create a problem with the external components of the cochlear implant system, extreme dryness with a buildup of static electricity can also present some difficulties. In classrooms that are very hot and dry, some simple precautions can be taken to help guard against problems caused by electrostatic discharge (ESD). Carpeting can be sprayed with a solution of 50% fabric softener and 50% water. If possible, humidifiers can also be placed in the classroom to increase the moisture.

On the playground, buildup of ESD when using plastic equipment, specifically slides, has generated concern. Children with cochlear implants should either remove their devices when using this equipment or should be counseled against playing on it. There have been some instances of map contamination or loss after playing on plastic apparatus. Since it is not a consistent finding, it is difficult to determine the exact combination of factors which may contribute to the problem. If a child has been in the playground, and suddenly exhibits changes in his functional ability with the implant, the teacher should notify the parent. The parent should be instructed to contact the implant facility to have the processor checked. Often, all that is required is a rewriting of the map to the speech processor.

■ TROUBLESHOOTING THE COCHLEAR IMPLANT SYSTEM

Parents and teachers should all have some exposure to methods that are used to troubleshoot the implant. The amount and type of exposure may depend on the implant facility servicing the child. At the very least, literature on how to perform these procedures should be made accessible. Booklets provided by the manufacturer are available on request. Additionally, some "hands-on" demonstration of troubleshooting techniques should be furnished. The educational consultant model lends itself to providing this type of training to teachers and therapists at local schools. Some centers (specifically the center at Manhattan Eye, Ear & Throat Hospital in New York) also provide a videotape of the troubleshooting procedures. If no communication between the school and the implant facility has occurred regarding this information, then the school should contact the facility and request it.

It should be acknowledged that the cochlear implant, like many other mechanical devices, will, at some point, not function properly or cease to function completely. It is important that teachers and therapists realize that they should not panic if this happens. Knowledge of how the system works will allow for troubleshooting the unit quickly and efficiently. It is important to remember that there can be more than one piece of equipment which is not functioning properly. Therefore, once a problem is found with one component, the troubleshooting process should continue to ensure the entire mechanism is functioning. Complete troubleshooting guides for both the Nucleus and the Clarion are found in Appendixes F and G, respectively. The following description relates to the Nucleus device only.

The flashing of the red display light on the top of the speech processor in response to speech indicates that the cochlear implant is functioning properly. (This should not be confused with the rhythmic flashing of the lights which signals low battery voltage.) A flashing light, in tandem with speech, only occurs when the unit is in the "N" or "S" position, the sensitivity is turned up to #3 or above and there is speech input into the microphone. If this light fails to flash, there is a problem with some portion of the external equipment. One method of testing the integrity of the entire external implant system requires the removal of the unit from the child. Once the unit is removed and can be easily visualized, the external transmitter (circular portion) is placed on the speech processor on the side that is marked with the name "Cochlear" (see Figure 6–6). If the unit is functioning properly, the two red display lights on the top of the speech processor should flash when vocalizing into the microphone. If these two red lights do not signal simultaneously, then there is a problem.

Also available from Cochlear Corporation is a piece of equipment known as the "wand." This wand allows the unit to be tested in the manner noted above, while the child is still wearing the device. The wand looks similar to the external transmitter with the exception of a small red light located in its center. When the wand is placed over the transmitter, this red light will glow if the unit is functioning properly.

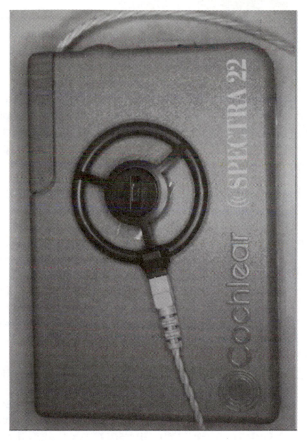

Figure 6–6
Placement of external transmitter over the speech processor.

Many educators prefer the "wand" as a method of quickly checking the unit without having to disturb the child.

If the unit fails to light (using either the wand or the child's own transmitter), there are a number of simple procedures that the teacher/therapist can use to troubleshoot the system. The first is to ensure that the unit is in the "N" or "S" position with the sensitivity turned up to its adjusted setting. (If this is unknown, the sensitivity dial should be set to #3 and tested at that setting). If the speech processor has erroneously been set on "T," only one of the red lights will be continuously lit. The next step is to ensure that all of the connections are making proper contact. The long cord, which extends from the microphone to the speech processor unit, should be plugged in at the base of the microphone so that the dot on the cord matches the dot on the microphone. If these two dots do not match, this may be the cause of the problem. Turning the cord so that the dots do match should restore the display lights to the normal flashing state if this is the only site of the problem. In addition to the long cord, the short cord from the microphone to the transmitter should be checked to ensure it is making proper contact. If both cords appear to be appropriate and the lights still do not glow, the next portion of the unit to check is the battery.

The battery may be a rechargeable or a standard alkaline. The teacher/therapist should make certain that the positive and negative poles of the battery are in the proper position and the battery fits snugly into its compartment. It is helpful if the child or classroom teacher has a spare battery so that a new one can be placed in the unit to determine if the battery is the problem. Even if the battery was inserted that day, it should always be replaced. (Rechargeable batteries last approximately 12 to 15 hours depending on device setting. Standard alkaline batteries are usually changed every other day. Battery life for the new Spectra processor is somewhat shorter for both types of batteries.) If, after changing the battery, the display lights begin to flash, the problem has been identified. If they do not flash, the next portion of the unit to change is the cords.

The school and/or child should always have a spare set of cords available for this purpose. The long cord should be exchanged first. If this does not correct the problem, the short cord should be replaced next. If the lights still fail to glow, the problem may be either in the microphone or the speech processor. To troubleshoot the microphone portion of the cochlear implant system, it is necessary to use the hand-held microphone which is part of the cochlear implant accessory kit. Often, teachers use this microphone as a means of direct input to the speech processor. Should the child's ear level microphone malfunction, the plug-in microphone can be used temporarily by fastening it to the child's lapel. If the teacher does not have access to the accessory microphone, then the parent should assume responsibility for this portion of the troubleshooting at home. When the problem is determined to be with the speech processor, the cochlear implant center must be contacted.

Often teachers ask, "If the processor is not working, should it be left on the child?" It is recommended that the device be worn by the child in the "off" position even if it is not functioning so that the unit is not lost or exposed to damaging situations. (For example, removing the unit and placing it the child's backpack might subject it to abuse from other materials in the backpack.) As long as the speech processor is in the "off" position, the child can continue to wear the nonfunctioning unit with no possibility of danger to the child or the unit.

■□ CONTRAINDICATIONS

There are a number of situations both medical and environmental which should be avoided after implantation. Medically, implant recipients may not be evaluated using Magnetic Resonance Imaging (MRI) since the internal receiver contains a magnet and physical damage may result. Any other type of X-ray procedure will not be problematic. Implant patients should always inform physicians that they have a cochlear implant. Should the individual require any other type of surgery, it is important that the implanting surgeon be advised.

Implant users should be aware of possible interference from two-way radios or cellular telephones which may operate on the same frequency. Airport security systems may be activated due to the presence of the implant magnet. If security personnel require that the speech processor be placed through the X-ray system, it will not cause any damage. If there are any other circumstances about which the parent or teacher is concerned, the implant center should be contacted.

■□ INTERNAL RECEIVER PROBLEMS

There are some instances when the external equipment is operating appropriately, but the child's auditory responsiveness has deteriorated or is suddenly inconsistent. Although there are a number of circumstances which might account for this behavior (e.g., a map change), there is also a small possibility there may be a problem with the functioning of the internal receiver. Cochlear Corporation has reported that the cumulative survival rate (i.e., the percentage of implants which survive during the course of the lifetime of a patient) for both adults and children in the United States is 98%. However, this rate drops to 93% when reviewing the pediatric population separately (Cochlear Corporation, 1993). The failure rate is reported to be the highest in males below the age of 6 years. Since analysis of failed receivers identified the antenna as the site of some of the breakdowns, changes to this portion of the internal receiver have been made. It is believed that this change should markedly reduce the percentage of failures in children.

Nonetheless, it is important for teachers and therapists to be aware of some of the "red flags" which may indicate a problem with the internal receiver. As stated previously, children whose performance suddenly deteriorates or those who are "consistently inconsistent" despite functioning external equipment, should be referred to the implant center for further testing. If children report that the signal is intermittent or there suddenly appears noise that cannot be eliminated with a change of equipment, then these children should also be referred. Children who have changed more than three pieces of equipment in a 1-month period should be considered at risk. Finally, if a child is not progressing according to the general trends that have been outlined by the educational consultant, suspicion should be raised regarding the functioning of the internal receiver.

Teachers or therapists suspecting a problem should not alarm the parents unnecessarily but should urge them to bring the child to the implant facility for further evaluation. Constant communication with the cochlear implant center concerning children who display any of the risk factors is critical for these youngsters.

■ TESTING THE SPEECH PROCESSOR BEHAVIORALLY

Teachers, therapists, and parents find checking the implant at the start of every day will prevent problems, especially for young children who may not be sophisticated wearers. Once children are able to respond consistently to speech signals, detection (or identification) of the Ling 6 sounds can be performed quickly to ascertain functioning of the device. The classroom teacher should not presume that the processor is working even if the parent has tested the system before the child left for school. Problems with any type of mechanical equipment can arise at any time. Therefore, it behooves the classroom teacher to check the equipment whenever there is deviation from the known baseline behavior on the part of the child. In the long term, a few minutes devoted to equipment check at the beginning of the day can circumvent hours of inattention or confusion on the part of the child.

■⊐ SUMMARY

Management of the child with a cochlear implant need not be clouded in the mystique and fear that tends to come with new technology. Teachers and therapists can provide input to the parents regarding device functioning by reporting any deviation to the family and/or implant center. Knowledge of the child's abilities at the time of the initial tune-up will assist the teacher and therapist in designing an immediate therapeutic plan. The most important consideration in providing good management for a child with an implant is the school personnel's ability to be as knowledgeable as possible in all aspects of implantation. This knowledge base is best provided through a combination of interactions with the implant facility and information from the parents. These numerous interactions will lead to successful management of a child with a cochlear implant.

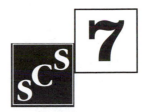

Premises that Drive Auditory Learning for Children with Cochlear Implants

Encouraging deaf children to use their residual hearing to develop listening skills has a long-standing history for educators committed to an oral approach in teaching the deaf. The degree to which audition is to be supplemented by other sensory modalities has been debated by many. Strict auditory verbal therapists withhold visual or tactile information from children for the purpose of encouraging dependence on auditory information. Educators employing a multisensory approach supplement auditory information with visual and tactile cues. Regardless of the presence or absence of additional sensory cues, the foundation of any auditory approach is the selection and fitting of the most appropriate listening device.

◧ SENSORY DEVICES

Prior to the availability of cochlear implants, the use of carefully selected hearing aids was considered the first step in designing a (re)habilitation program. Historically, body aids were the workhorses of hearing aid technology. The profoundly deaf child needed maximal power to amplify sound to a perceptible level. Advances in hearing aid design, especially miniaturization, led to the widespread acceptance of behind-the-ear hearing aids for even the profoundly deaf child. Frequency modulation devices (FM devices) reduce ambient noise in the classroom by providing input from a teacher's microphone directly to the child via FM radio signal. Using FM systems requires the child to wear a body unit which is either attached to earmolds or "booted" to behind the ear aids. This unit receives the signal from the teacher's microphone and transmits it to the ear. FMs have generally been used as classroom amplification systems; however, because of their increased power output potential a small number of profoundly deaf children use FM systems as personal hearing aids.

Relying on the technology of hearing aids alone meant that some profoundly deaf children with little or no measurable hearing were left without access to sound. Even when fit with the most powerful amplification possible, these children were not able to respond with hearing aids. Boothroyd (1982) suggested that children with total or near total losses had access to sound only through the sense of touch. Because touch conveys time and intensity information, it could be used to help children recognize sound with some characteristic patterns, such as some environmental sounds. With regard to the perception of speech, Boothroyd predicted that only about a 10 to 15% improvement in speechreading could be attributed to providing supplemental tactile stimulation. Nevertheless, even this minimal contribution to improving communication ability was considered to be an asset. Thus, a number of children with total losses were fit with vibrotactile devices. Vibrotactile devices convert sound into vibrations that can be felt on the skin. Early devices presented all speech sounds into a single oscillator; more sophisticated devices attempted to provide frequency information by using multiple oscillators. Despite special training to help individuals interpret tactile information as auditory (Eilers, Vergara, Cobo-Lewis, & Oller, 1994; Plant, 1989), performance with vibrotactile devices has been problematic due to the contamination of the speech signal with extraneous noise. Many of the results indicating good use of vibrotactile information have been obtained under ideal listening conditions. Profoundly deaf children who made modest gains with the vibrotactile aid are now one of the target populations for cochlear implants. In fact, many implant facilities utilize vibrotactile stimulation as part of the pre-implant evaluation process. Cochlear implant technology enables the profoundly deaf to have more access to auditory information than is possible through either hearing aids or vibrotactile devices. The development of auditory skills is now a reasonable expectation for the profoundly deaf child with an implant.

At this point, the important relationship between listening skills and the development of speech skills must be introduced. It has long been a fact that a reciprocal-type relationship exists between hearing ability and speech production. The more significant the hearing loss, the less likely the deaf child is to develop intelligible speech. Research has shown that children with significant residual hearing have a better chance at developing good speech intelligibility (Boothroyd, 1976; Hudgins & Numbers, 1942). It is believed that the increased auditory capability provided by the cochlear implant enables profoundly deaf children to achieve better speech perception and, as a byproduct, develop more intelligible speech. Indeed, there is now evidence to support the implant's effects on both speech perception and production of profoundly deaf children (Geers and Moog, 1991; Osberger et al., 1991a; Staller et al., 1991).

■□ AUDITORY TRAINING SKILLS
IN PROFESSIONALS

Methods and procedures for developing auditory skills in deaf children were historically taught in teacher preparation programs as part of the Speech Development course or the course in Aural Rehabilitation. The rise of Total Communication has caused training programs to add a sign language component to the already full college curriculum. Because of this, information about audition, or the role of auditory input for the development of speech and spoken language, is likely to be de-emphasized. Responsibilities for the development of these aspects of language have been relegated to the speech-language pathologist or educational audiologist. This is problematic due to the limited coursework focusing on the habilitation of young deaf children at the graduate level in speech-language pathology programs. Moreover, educational audiology is a specialty still in its infancy, and the number of trained educational audiologists is relatively small (Medwetsky, 1994).

It is the classroom teacher who is still the most knowledgeable professional regarding the skills and abilities of deaf children. Yet, teachers are seldom taught how to enhance audition in these youngsters. In addition, a number of teacher preparation programs have identified themselves as Bilingual/Bicultural programs. This means that they teach ASL and support the cultural model of deafness. It is likely that preservice teachers in these programs will have no exposure to the issues of speech, spoken language, or audition at all; these are an anathema to the "Bi/Bi" approach.

■□ FROM AUDITORY TRAINING TO AUDITORY LEARNING

Preservice or graduate teacher preparation programs that value audition and the development of speech and spoken language continue to train professionals to develop listening skills in deaf children. Although many of the basic tenets of auditory speech perception remain the same, the philosophical orientation for the development of auditory skills in deaf children has shifted markedly. No longer is the deaf child taught to learn *to* listen, but to learn *through* listening. This belief dictates a thorough understanding of the principles of auditory *learning* rather than auditory *training*.

Auditory training called for listening practice in small group activities. Often these lessons began with the discrimination of nonverbal sounds such as bells, drums, and whistles. Listening to speech occurred only after success in identifying these gross noisemakers. Ling (1986) suggested that auditory training results were seldom satisfactory because the training rarely related to the child's speech and spoken language development, cognitive level, or everyday life experiences. Mischook and Cole (1986) described auditory learning as "the normal development of a synergistic cluster composed of auditory, speech and language abilities" (p. 69). They further recommended that auditory learning be best accomplished through "natural, enjoyable intervention."

■□ AUDITORY LEARNING AND COCHLEAR IMPLANTS

Experience suggests that the age of the individual at the time of implantation dictates whether a listening program is *re*habilitative or habilitative. That is, does it emphasize training or learning? Certainly the adult implant user or the child who is postlinguistically deafened can benefit from training or practice with drill-like materials to re-establish auditory pathways for processing sound. On the other hand, children implanted at a young age (between the ages of 2 and 4), will more likely benefit from placement in an environment in which listening has meaning and is required for completing tasks of interest. The overall habilitation goal for children in this group is the development of language. Building communicative competence is the highest priority for the young deaf child. It is probable, however, that there is merit to providing these same youngsters with some opportunity to participate in activities in which *listening* is the focus of the language-driven task. These "lessons" should not be decontextualized and rote. Parents and teachers who create games which practice listening skills, while at the same time provide quality social (or academic) interaction, may accelerate the child's acquisition of auditory skills.

■□ BASIC TASKS OF AUDITORY SPEECH PERCEPTION

Hearing impairment reduces the amount of auditory information available to be processed by the brain. Once the information, however reduced, gets to the brain, there are four levels of processing which can occur. The most simplistic level of processing, *detection*, is the awareness that a sound has been made. The most complex level, *comprehension*, requires both the perception of sound and knowledge of language to interpret that sound. Between these two extremes are the auditory skills of *discrimination* and *identification* (Erber, 1982).

The ultimate goal of listening practice is always auditory comprehension or understanding through listening. It must be acknowledged, however, that the development of auditory skills is always framed in a language context. Therefore, the linguistic/auditory relationship must be understood in order to interpret performance in the auditory domain. A child who has a rudimentary sign/speech vocabulary may not be able to participate in listening tasks that require more language understanding. The listening *ability* may be present, but it will remain untapped because the constraints of the linguistic system will not allow it to be assessed. Further, the relationship between listening to and producing speech must be established at the inception of auditory work. Ideas for building these relationships will be presented in the discussion of the Premises.

Detection

Demonstrating that a sound has been detected requires that the listener, in some way, indicate that it has been heard. It is not necessary for the child to identify the sound in order to be rated as having detected it. It is necessary, however, for him to respond within a certain time limit once a stimulus has been presented. A timely response is required in order to tell the difference between a slow and uncertain response to a presented stimulus and a definite "no" response to the absence of a stimulus. The teachers/therapists must create a listening "window" for the child. This "window" establishes a time for the youngster to listen for and respond to the presence (or absence) of a stimulus. For example, the child may be asked to listen for his name and say "yes" when the teacher says his name and "no" if the teacher says nothing. After teaching the task in a looking and listening trial, the teacher covers her mouth, presents the child's name in an auditory-only trial, and looks expectantly at the child to respond appropriately. The teacher presents the child's name again, waits, and the child responds appropriately by saying "yes." Before presenting the third listening set, the teacher pauses to have the child wait for the stimulus. However, in this trial, there is no stimulus presented. The teacher uncovers her mouth and looks to the child to respond. In this presentation, the proper response from the child is "no." Incorporating the concept of the listening window requires a response after every trial regardless of whether a stimulus is actually presented.

Speech Versus Environmental Sounds

When asked to detect a sound, it is not necessary for the child to tell whether it is a speech sound or an environmental sound. Speech sounds could be a single sound (/sh/), a nonsense syllable (a two or three letter syllable that is not a real word, e.g., bah), a child's name, a phrase, or a sentence. Environmental sounds are those sounds which are produced all around us that are not speech-like. These include a microwave oven timer, the telephone, a car horn, or a lawnmower. A child with a cochlear implant is most likely to demonstrate the skill of detection soon after the speech processor is activated (see Chapter 6, Initial Responses after Tune-Up). Initially, the parent or teacher may want to alert the child to sounds that are occurring or about to occur. This gives the child the opportunity to focus his attention for a specific listening interval rather than constantly scanning his environment auditorally. (The ability to scan the environment and detect sounds independently is a more mature response and will develop after some experience with listening.)

A child may demonstrate detection by searching for the source of the sound or he may look inquisitively at the teacher or parent as if to ask, "Did I hear something?" He may ask simply "What was that?" or he may imitate it (as in a speech sound or the "beep, beep, beep" of the microwave). In still other circumstances, the child may stop participating in an activity in which he was engaged. Particular examples of the variety of *active* responses which would indicate that a child has detected a speech sound include clapping after hearing the sounds of the 6-Sound test in an auditory only presentation; looking up from a book when the blocks crash on the floor in the play area; or turning when he hears a teacher's or parent's voice saying his name, "STOP!" or "NO! NO!" in a quiet environment.

Discrimination

Processing auditory information at the level of discrimination does not require that the child label the sound heard. Once again, sound could be speech, speech-like, or environmental. To demonstrate discrimination ability, a listener need only indicate that two presented sounds were either the same or different. Discrimination tasks are generally more contrived than detection tasks and must be planned by the teacher or parent. A discrimination task requires that the teacher or parent say two words or two short sentences and ask the child to make the same/different judgment. Particular examples of discrimination tasks and the responses that might be expected from the child can be found below:

Example 1: Pictures and Response Cards

Directions: Using pictures to support directions and response cards to serve as an aid to clarifying the child's answer, the parent teaches the task. Response cards are constructed with pictures which represent the abstract concept same/different, for example, one card could have two pictures or stickers that are the same and one card could show two different pictures or stickers. If the child uses total communication, then direction should be given in sign. However listening stimuli are always presented without sign support.

(continued)

Teacher/Parent:	I will be talking about names of people in the family. I will say two names; maybe I will say the same name two times or two different names. You will have to tell me if the names are the same or different. Or, you can point to *this* picture if they are the same, and *this* picture if they are different. These are the names I will use: Mom, Uncle Bill. Let's practice first with looking and listening. MOM, UNCLE BILL. Did I say two names that were the same or two different names?
Child:	Two different names (or child points to the appropriate card).
Teacher/Parent:	Good. Let's try with listening only. MOM, MOM. Same or different?
Child:	Same.
Teacher/Parent:	That's right. Listen again.

As the child becomes more sophisticated, new names can be added to the list. Initially, the patterns of the names should be dissimilar to insure that the differences can be detected. These patterns can be made more similar as the child's level of response improves. Same/different judgments can also be made using sentence material for children whose language ability can support it.

	Example 2: Sentences
Teacher/Parent:	I'm going to say two things from our list of school senten-ces. Let's look at all the sentences first:
	It's time for speech.
	(continued)

Get your lunchbox.

What is the weather today?

How many children came to school?

Here are two sentences that I will say. Maybe I will say one of them twice or maybe I will say each one of them once—Get your lunchbox. How many children came to school? You need to look and listen and tell me if the two sentences that I say are the same or different. GET YOUR LUNCHBOX. HOW MANY CHILDREN CAME TO SCHOOL? Were those sentences the same or different?

Child: They were different.

Parent/Teacher: Yes, that's what I said. Let's try with listening only.

Included in these brief examples were a number of key instructional strategies which were overlaid onto the dialogue. These strategies serve as the foundation for planning effective auditory activities. First and foremost, the teacher/parent explains the task carefully so that she is sure the child knows what to do. Before presenting him with the actual listening task, the teacher reviews the stimuli in the closed set (i.e., all the possible answers). He is given a number of opportunities to demonstrate the ability to perform the task in a looking and listening trial. (In the examples above, only one trial was demonstrated for illustrative purposes.) His response in these trials indicates that he is capable of performing the task. If the child then fails to perform the task when it is presented in an auditory-only mode, it may be assumed that the task is beyond his auditory capability. It should also be noted that in discrimination tasks, regardless of the whether the child is listening to a word or a sentence, he is only required to make a same/different response.

Identification

In tasks of auditory identification, a child is asked to listen to one item, presented from a group of similar items (defined above as a closed set) and choose the one presented. This choice can be indicated in any one of a number of ways: by pointing to items or pictures representing the items, through manipulating (picking up or throwing) an item named or through repetition of what was heard. As with discrimination tasks, identification tasks can be planned using any one of a number of materials based on the linguistic development and auditory needs of the child. Thus, he may be asked to identify speech sounds, words, phrases, sentences, or connected sentences. Particular examples of listening tasks at different language levels and the closed sets that the teacher/ parent may arrange include:

Example 3: Speech Sounds

Teacher/Parent:	We are going to practice listening to some of our speech sounds. These are all the sounds that I might say: bah, boo, bee, boe. Let's says them together.
Teacher and Child:	bah, boo, bee, boe
Teacher/Parent:	Good. Now you watch and listen and I will say a sound and you tell me which one I said. BEE
Child:	bee
Teacher/Parent:	Yes, that's what I said. Now let's try with listening only. BOE. Which sound did I say?
Child:	boe
Teacher/Parent:	That's right. Listen again.

(continued)

Example 4 : Words

Teacher/Parent: We have been talking about things that go. Here is a truck, an airplane and a submarine. You tell me the name of the one that I point to (Teacher is ensuring that the child knows the vocabulary).

Child: airplane, truck, submarine

Teacher/Parent: I will tell you one word and you make the toy move. First we will try with looking and listening. Then we will try with listening only. Ready. SUBMARINE

Child: (moves the submarine across the table)

Teacher/Parent: Good. Now you listen and I will tell you which one to move. TRUCK.

Child: (drives truck across the table)

Teacher/Parent: Yes, I said truck. Now let's try again.

Example 5: Sentences

Teacher/Parent: Here is our story from the day we made pudding. Who remembers that day? OK, Let's read our story together. Then we will listen to the sentences. You can point to the sentence on the chart. Then you can take a turn being the teacher.

(continued)

Teacher and Child: We made chocolate pudding.
Colleen poured the milk into the bowl.
Bobby mixed and mixed the pudding.
Everyone liked the pudding except Kate.

Teacher/Parent: I will tell you one sentence and you show me on the chart which sentence I said. Ready. You can watch and listen first. BOBBY MIXED AND MIXED THE PUDDING.

Child: (points to sentence on chart and "reads" it)

Teacher/Parent: Good. Now this time, let's just listen. WE MADE CHOCOLATE PUDDING.

Child: (points to correct sentence and repeats the sentence)

Teacher/Parent: Yes, that's what I said. Now let's try another one. You can be the teacher now.

Example 6: Connected Sentences (Nursery Rhymes)

Teacher/Parent: We have been listening to nursery rhymes. Who can tell me one nursery rhyme we know?

Child: Jack and Jill

Teacher/Parent: Yes, Jack and Jill is one we know. Let's say it together.

Teacher and Child: Jack and Jill went up the hill to fetch a pail of water.
Jack fell down and broke his crown and Jill came tumbling after.

Can anyone think of another rhyme we know?

(continued)

Child:	We know Twinkle, Twinkle
Teacher/Parent:	Yes, that is a nursery song. Let's say it together.
Teacher and Child:	Twinkle, twinkle little star, How I wonder what you are Up above the world so high, Like a diamond in the sky Twinkle, twinkle little star, How I wonder what you are.
Teacher/Parent:	Can anyone think of one more?
Child:	Mary Had a Little Lamb
Teacher/Parent:	Yes, that's correct! Let's say the first part all together.
Teacher and Child:	Mary had a little lamb Its fleece was white as snow And everywhere that Mary went The lamb was sure to go.
Teacher/Parent:	Good. Now we have three rhymes that we are going to be listening for. But I will only say one. Listen to the whole rhyme before you make your choice. (teacher says the rhyme Jack and Jill)
Child:	(points to picture of Jack and Jill)
Teacher/Parent:	That's right. I said the Jack and Jill rhyme. Good listening. Now you try one and I will listen.

Through discussion of the auditory skill of identification, another key principle of preparing auditory activities is suggested: The linguistic level of the materials used should become increasingly complex if the child's language abilities can support it. All activities outlined provide practice in the skill of closed set identification; the level of language at which the skill is practiced is determined by the linguistic abilities of the child. Not only is the activity itself driven by the language level of the child, but the directions for participating in the activity must be within the child's language ability.

Comprehension

The most sophisticated level of listening demonstrates auditory comprehension of language. Robbins (1994) refers to this skill as a "thinking while listening" task. When a child is asked to think while listening, he must make a judgment or decision about what was heard and produce a verbal response which is more than just the repetition of the stimulus. The response can be a member of a closed set, but, more often, it is a new response that is the result of comprehending what was heard. For example, based on Nevins et al. (1991), the teacher presents a child with a set of mixed vocabulary words and the task is to choose the one that does not belong (teacher presents VOLCANOES, COLONIST, DESERT, MOUNTAINS. The child responds COLONIST, because it is a social studies vocabulary word and the others are science words). In another example, the teacher may ask the child to respond with the opposite of a word presented (teacher presents TALL and the child responds SHORT) or think of words that are associated with another word (teacher presents RAIN and child responds UMBRELLA).

At a more complex linguistic level, a child may be asked to respond to a question: Who mixed the pudding? (from the earlier experience story, the response would be "Bobby"); state whether a given sentence is true or false: Colleen poured applesauce into the bowl (this sentence is false, Colleen poured *milk* into the bowl); or complete the rhyme, Jack fell down and broke his crown . . . (and Jill came tumbling after).

The thinking while listening task represents a higher order auditory skill and is one that is often overlooked. Teachers must seize opportunities which require even those children with limited language abilities to listen at this level. The cochlear implant creates the possibility for more children to achieve comprehension of auditory input.

■ THE PREMISES

Individuals who approach the task of postimplant habilitation should have a knowledge base and a rationale for applying that knowledge. A fully articulated set of principles which guides all of the recommendations set forth in this and subsequent chapters is offered as the foundation on which specific auditory activities can be developed. These premises are the result of discussions among the cochlear implant team members at the Manhattan Eye, Ear & Throat Hospital and reflect a blending of individual philosophies and personal experiences with deaf children using cochlear implants.

Premise One

The development of speech perception and speech production abilities is the primary goal of implantation. Therefore, meaningful speech should be used as the input for listening tasks.

As indicated earlier, traditional auditory training curricula often begin skill development with the detection, discrimination, and identification of gross and environmental sounds. This is accomplished by sounding musical instruments, activating appliances which make noise, or playing an audio recording of either or both. Although the signal processors of both the Nucleus and the Clarion devices will deliver environmental sound information to the electrode array, their main purpose is to process speech. Therefore, providing listening practice for nonspeech stimuli does not take full advantage of the processors' abilities. Further, the importance of context in helping a child learn through listening cannot be overstated. Removing environmental sounds from their normal context and presenting them in a classroom setting violates the concept of the natural environment.

The child should be encouraged to respond to environment sounds which occur naturally in home and at school. At home, the telephone, microwave, vacuum cleaner, and doorbell are all appropriate targets for detection and identification of these sounds. Environmental sounds which naturally occur in or around the classroom/school setting include the dismissal bell, intercom system, fire alarm, lawnmower and, in some cases, a telephone in the classroom. Teachers/therapists should always reinforce the child's response to sound. However, the focus of structured practice for listening should be meaningful speech.

The form of this "meaningful speech" is dictated by the language level of the child. This is not to suggest, however, that there is a simplistic building block phenomenon when it comes to providing auditory and linguistic input to the child. By integrating the theories of top-down and bottom-up processing (Paterson, 1986), the teacher/therapist plans listening activities which utilize both small and large units of meaningful speech (e.g., words, sentences, or connected sentences). More importantly, listening to small units of meaningful speech (words) should not be abandoned as a child becomes increasingly advanced linguistically. There is continued merit to using words for listening practice, especially when acoustic information about those words varies. For example, word stimuli can be presented which range from very different ("fruit" vs. "vegetables"), to similar ("orange" vs. "cherry"), to very similar ("cherry" vs. "berry").

Premise Two

The goal of any listening activity includes the activation of the speech/auditory feedback loop. Therefore, listening practice should always provide an opportunity for a productive response.

As listening skills are developed during the postimplant period, it is critically important that the child see the relationship between listening and speaking. What we hear shapes what we say. Children need to learn about the existence of this relationship so that they can use their newfound listening ability to improve speech production. However, in many published auditory training curricula, listening practice is accomplished by setting up choices for the child that require a pointing response: I heard "this" (child points to picture) or I heard "that" (child points to word). In this situation, the child may conclude that listening is an activity separate from talking. Training listening skills in isolation, without linking them to speech and spoken language, may result in *compartmentalized* development. One way to avoid compartmentalization is to pair auditory tasks with a spoken language response. Although pairing auditory tasks to a spoken response is not a new concept, it is common to expect nonverbal responses in traditional auditory evaluation tasks. For example, a large number of auditory tests do not require the child to speak to indicate a response. In soundfield testing, conditioned play audiometry is nonverbal in nature. The older child also makes nonverbal responses to test tones. Even speech perception and auditory comprehension tests such as the Word Intelligibility by Picture Identification (WIPI) (Ross & Lerman, 1971) or the Test of Auditory Comprehension (TAC) (Trammell et al., 1981) accept a pointing response. A nonverbal response is particularly necessary when testing the listening abilities of profoundly deaf children. Examiners do not wish to confound the results of perception testing by trying to understand what may be unintelligible speech; but, this is a testing paradigm and one that is not appropriate for teaching.

Listening activities that are built on a testing paradigm may continue a pattern of nonverbal response. It is recommended, therefore, that a child be required to make a *productive response* when participating in listening tasks. Given this belief, a child should always be made to respond to a stimulus by either repeating it, responding to a question, or taking a turn to be the teacher. If the listening task is differentiating between a one syllable word and a two syllable word (and recall that a child need not identify the word, but can accomplish this task based solely on pattern perception) the teacher/therapist can ask the child to repeat the stimulus. The goal is for the child to demonstrate that he can produce a single beat approximation of the word or a two beat approximation. He must evidence that his ability to *hear* the pattern difference has carried over to his ability to *produce* this difference.

The same perception/production relationship holds true for more complex input. If a child can demonstrate that he hears the difference between a short sentence and a long sentence (WE WENT TO THE ZOO and WE SAW MANY MONKEYS AT THE MONKEY HOUSE) or a sentence with an exclamation in it versus a simple declarative sentence (HOORAY! WE SAW A SEA LION SHOW vs. THE GIRAFFES HAD REALLY LONG NECKS), he should also be encouraged to differentiate production of these sentence pairs. Planning activities that require a productive response can help to assure the teacher that important speech/listening ties are being established.

Accepting this premise is particularly important for the teachers and parents of children who use total communication. It is easy to accept a productive *sign* response rather than a productive *speech* response. Teachers and parents are reminded that the important speech/listening link must be made both at home and at school so that the expectation of spoken language from the child is supported by all.

Premise Three

There are certain cognitive and linguistic precursors that are necessary for successful auditory work.

All tasks presented to children require that they understand what it is they are supposed to do (cognitive precursor) and the language that is used to tell them what to do (linguistic precursor). When a child performs a task auditorally, it is assumed that he understands the nature of the task and the language used to complete it. For a child who is unable to perform a task auditorally, the possibility exists that a language problem is preventing him from responding appropriately. To rule out a problem with language, the teacher/therapist can present the stimulus a second time, adding visual clues (lipreading and/or signing) to determine if the child is successful under these conditions. If he is, it can then be assumed that he has sufficient linguistic skills to complete the task. His inability to perform in an auditory-only modality suggests that he has reached a ceiling in his auditory skills at the present time. If, however, the child cannot perform the task when given both auditory and visual information, it may be inferred that the directions of the activity are too difficult for him to understand. It may also be the case that unfamiliarity with the language and vocabulary of the task prevents him from responding appropriately. To ascertain the source of difficulty, the teacher/therapist first simplifies the language of the directions and repeats the activity. Should this fail, she simplifies the language of the stimulus and presents it again, in an audition-plus-vision condition. If the child is then successful, the teacher/therapist can present the task auditorally only with the confidence that she is truly tapping auditory, not language, ability.

When simplifying the language fails to help the child respond successfully to the task, given both auditory and visual cues, the teacher may question if the child understands what is expected. Modeling the type of response required and providing assistance to the child in performing the task are useful strategies for dealing with this problem. Additionally, modifying the activity so that the child can be successful by performing an alternate task can also be helpful. It is imperative that the child demonstrate both understanding of the task and understanding of the language before the teacher makes a judgment about auditory ability based on failure to respond.

These issues may appear to be self-evident when the child in question is young and his understanding of language and school-like tasks is still developing. It is often erroneously assumed that older children understand the language and the tasks set before them. Indeed, deaf children are often afraid to indicate that they have not understood or, perhaps, are unaware that they have not. They will often respond positively to the question "Do you understand?" when, in fact, they are uncertain about what is expected. A child's error response to an auditory task must be rigorously analyzed, as must the tasks themselves, in order to interpret a child's auditory abilities fairly and accurately.

Premise Four

Cochlear implants will likely provide all children with supraseg-mental speech cues. Others may have auditory access to segmental speech information. Regardless, the ability to benefit from the implant can be sharpened with specific listening practice.

Experience to date suggests that the cochlear implant provides a measure of auditory ability that the child did not have prior to implantation. However, it is not enough to implant a child and wait for listening skills simply to develop. Focused listening practice will likely enhance and accelerate the benefit an individual can receive from the device (Tye-Murray & Fryauf-Bertschy, 1992). Earlier, the concept of auditory learning was introduced. The statements reflected in this premise are not meant to undermine that idea. Although the provision of an environment for auditory learning is necessary, it is likely insufficient for the development of many of the auditory skills made possible with the implant. The ability to detect the patterns of speech or the *suprasegmental* aspects of speech is one of the auditory skills which develops soon after implantation. *Suprasegmental* is defined as above the level of individual sounds and includes rhythm, intonation and stress patterns. On the other hand, *segmental* information is conveyed by individual sounds. For example, if a child hears the difference between the words "bit" and "bat," he does so because he hears the difference between the individual sounds "i" and "a." He is relying on segmental information for this discrimination. If the child hears the difference between the words "bat" and "baseball" and can indicate that they are not the same, he has done so, at the very least, by relying on suprasegmental information. In this case, the suprasegmental information is pattern information. The word "bat" is a one syllable word and the word "baseball" is a two syllable word. Differentiating between two words on the basis of patterns, or more specifically, suprasegmental information, is a task appropriate for a newly implanted child.

Pattern perception encompasses more than just syllable numbers in words. Pattern information aids in distinguishing between sentences as well. Suprasegmental information contributes to the difference between the sentences, "Get your lunchbox" and "After we eat lunch we will play outside." In this example, the suprasegmental information is carried by sentence length.

Pattern perception can be helpful in discriminating between two sentences. It can also be used to recognize certain auditory patterns which convey specific information, for example, the pattern of direct address in a classroom setting. This pattern is characterized by a one, two, or three syllable word (the child's name) followed by a brief pause and then the remainder of the sentence (e.g., Amy, time to go to Speech). Children should be alerted to this pattern and encouraged to "scan the auditory environment" periodically to listen for it. This configuration suggests that a name is being called and a direction given. Although the child at the level of this auditory perceptual skill cannot understand the exact message through listening only, he is signaled by the pattern that a name is being called. He can look up to focus his attention on the teacher and be ready for additional information.

Still another suprasegmental pattern which may be important for the child in a classroom is the pattern which signals seriation. This pattern is characterized by a short string of connected words followed by individual words separated by pauses. It suggests that a list is being presented (It's time for Math; you need your pencils, your workbooks, your counters, and your numberline). A child should be taught to recognize this pattern as well. If he is aware of the "template" he can count the number of items between pauses. Coupling that with his knowledge of the routine, he can ascertain how many items to gather and make an educated guess as to which items are required for the lesson.

It cannot be expected that a child will learn these auditory patterns and discriminate among them in the context of the classroom. Thus, this premise advocates specific listening practice. However, the introduction and development of skills such as these in listening sessions are only practical if there is carryover into the classroom setting.

As a child with an implant masters more sophisticated levels of listening, the teacher/therapist can help the child develop listening skills which make use of segmental cues. For example, the phoneme "s" in the English language carries much linguistic information. It signals plurals, possessives, some contractions, verb tense, and number (e.g., The cats are playing. The cat's tail is long. That cat's got a ball to play with. The cat sleeps in the sun). Children can practice listening for this important phoneme and learn to interpret the meaning of its presence as part of a total auditory habilitation plan.

Premise Five

If classroom listening is one of the goals of auditory practice, it follows that the content of the auditory lesson be suggested by the child's classroom curriculum.

Adults were the first individuals to receive the cochlear implant; implantation in children came after success was demonstrated in the adult population. Rehabilitative materials developed for adults were largely drill and practice tasks based on the vocabulary and everyday sentences of the world of the adult. This model uses words and sentences in a generic rehabilitation program sufficiently general so that it is appropriate to everyone (although, perhaps, interesting to none). Unfortunately, some implant centers have adopted this training paradigm for their young adults or children with the device.

Children are far less homogeneous than adults when it comes to life experiences or language ability. Rather than attempt to find material simplistic enough so that it is adaptable to all children, it is suggested that a child's individual language and vocabulary inventory be the basis for the development of auditory tasks specific to that child. The content of these lessons can be derived from classroom material— from the 3-year-old's lesson on dressing appropriately for the weather to the adolescent's discussion of the deserts of the world. Not only does the child have an opportunity to practice listening, but he also engages in a vocabulary and fact review through the repeated exposure to his school instruction. Protocols for implementing the recommendations set forth in this premise are detailed in Chapters 8 and 9.

Premise Six

Listening practice should be provided with a variety of input units: the phoneme, the word, the phrase, or sentence and connected discourse.

Familiarity with the concepts of top-down and bottom-up processing is necessary in order to appreciate the significance of this premise. Comparing the listening task to the reading task may be helpful in understanding these processing terms. Reading specialists who view reading as a bottom-up process advocate for phonic-type approaches for instruction. In this approach, individual sounds are learned and associated with letters. The child is required to blend two or three letters to make a simple word. After a number of simple words are learned, they are put together to make rather simple (and sometimes simplistic) sentences, for example, Ann ran to Dan. Basic sentences combine to make stories. New letter combinations are learned to make more simple words, and the process begins again.

Advocates of top-down theories of reading suggest that children need not be concerned with individual sounds. In fact, all that is necessary is an understanding of the subject matter and some basic sight vocabulary. Children are asked to bring their world knowledge to the reading task and decipher the story's message through educated guesses. Thus, a child who is knowledgeable about life on a farm will more easily read and comprehend a story written about this setting than a child without this experience.

Those who are moderates in the field of reading believe that neither extreme represents an explanation of the task. It is more likely that some sort of interaction between top-down and bottom-up efforts contribute to learning to read successfully. Applying this concept to this premise likens listening to phonemes or individual sounds to the bottom-up approach to the development of reading ability. This would be tedious indeed, for although individual sounds do carry meaning (as in the case of the phoneme "s") no one speaks in individual sounds. Further, building a listening repertoire with a bottom-up approach could take forever. On the other hand, if a child is exposed only to running speech or connected sentences, it would be virtually impossible for him to choose the salient information in that discourse.

There is important suprasegmental information conveyed by connected sentences, however, that may only occur at the level of discourse. Differentiating between patterns that represent conversation (continuous connected sentences in which speakers alternate turns) versus a set of directions (a single speaker producing a series of sentences, each separated by a brief pause) require that connected discourse be the stimulus. Distinguishing conversation from directions may be critically important in transition periods between subjects in the self-contained classroom. If a child hears continuous connected sentences between two speakers it may indicate that a teacher is conversing with another student. This signals that auditory attention is not required at this time. However, the pattern of directions, a single speaker issuing multiple sentences, each separated by a brief pause, signals the need to attend. This alerts the child to be ready to hear a homework assignment or prepare for the start of the next subject.

Premise Seven

There is a complex relationship between language and listening skills.

All auditory tasks that use meaningful speech as the stimuli must be designed with the understanding of the interdependent relationship of language and listening skills. Erber (1982) identified six units of speech stimuli: speech elements (phoneme), syllables, words, phrases, sentences, and connected discourse. He suggested that nearly all tasks of speech perception to which a child is exposed can be placed into one of these categories. These must then be considered simultaneously with the four tasks of auditory speech perception: detection, discrimination, identification, and comprehension. Each auditory task must be paired with each language level in order to provide practice at each intersection of auditory/language ability. However, this suggests an auditory/linguistic relationship that overlooks the concept of the linguistic environment. The linguistic environment refers to the language context in which auditory targets are placed. Engineering the linguistic environment calls for increasing the complexity of the language that surrounds the auditory target. Thus, if the child is differentiating between the one syllable and three syllable fruit words, peach and banana, the target words are in isolation. Requiring that the child differentiate between these same two words when they appear in a sentence context makes the auditory task a bit more difficult. Asking the child to choose between "I like to eat a banana" and "I like to eat a peach" necessitates his filtering past the additional signals in the sentences to the target auditory task, discriminating between a one and three syllable word.

Teachers and clinicians must be cognizant of the concept of the linguistic environment in order to more fully prepare a child for real-life listening. Thus, once any particular listening skill is mastered at the phoneme or word or phrase level, that same skill must be practiced in increasingly complex linguistic environments. An additional feature that must be considered in managing the linguistic environment is the placement of the target word within the sentence. It is all too often the case that target words for listening contrasts are placed at the end of sentences. Teachers and clinicians must make a conscious effort to avoid overusing this pattern and attempt to present sentences in which target placement varies. Although these sentences may be somewhat contrived, the teacher who is aware of the auditory needs of her children may plan lessons to accommodate these auditory objectives.

Premise Eight

Tasks at the phoneme level should be selected by the teacher based on the analysis of the speech production errors made by the child.

Speech errors made by deaf children are innumerable. Often, a particular child's repertoire contains errors or error patterns that are idiosyncratic or individual to that particular child. These include errors of substitution of one sound for another: "b" for "m" as in "bike" for "Mike"; omission of sounds as in "ouse" for "house"; distortion of sounds as in a "cough" in place of a "k"; and the addition of sounds in words or phrases as in "bulue" for "blue." Traditionally teachers have relied on developmental sequences that suggest the order in which deaf children develop particular speech sounds (Calvert & Silverman, 1983; Ling, 1976). This premise suggests that teachers also listen to what a child is saying incorrectly and use his own speech errors as the basis for selecting speech goals. Experience to date suggests that children with cochlear implants do not follow the same sequence for the development of sounds that other deaf children follow. In fact, high frequency sounds (e.g., /s/ and /sh/), which are more difficult for the deaf child to master because of hearing aid limitations, may be among some of the earlier developing sounds for the child with an implant. Implant technology allows these sounds to be coded and delivered.

The teacher/clinician is also encouraged to use audition to develop new sounds or remediate those sounds in error. If, for example, in a discussion on pollution, the child says "polluchun," the teacher can do a minilesson on the production of the /sh/. The teacher can ask the child to listen to the correct pronunciation or contrast auditorally both the correct and incorrect productions. If the child can identify correct productions auditorally, then he should be encouraged to produce the sound himself.

Incorporating this premise calls for the teacher to be responsible for the production of good speech in the classroom. For strategies for the development of speech sounds and the correction of sounds produced in error, the reader is directed to classic texts such as *Speech and Deafness* (Calvert & Silverman, 1983) and *Speech: Theory and Practice for the Hearing-Impaired Child* (Ling, 1976). Teachers knowledgeable about speech development and who believe it is their responsibility to teach speech as well as language and subject matter may already be practicing the recommendation set forth in this premise.

■□ SUMMARY

The cochlear implant has made it possible for profoundly deaf children to gain access to the auditory signal. This technology has created a reawakening to many of the basic tenets of auditory-speech perception. Underlying premises which guide professionals charged with exploiting audition outline important elements of a comprehensive auditory learning curriculum. Creating a climate in which auditory learning can take place is the primary responsibility of the classroom teacher and therapist. Specific practice to acquire particular listening skills from detection to comprehension may be beneficial to the implant recipient as well. This practice may accelerate overall auditory growth if it is based on the premises presented.

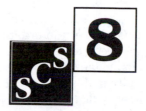

The Young
Implant Recipient

Currently, the lowest age limit for the implantation of profoundly deaf children is 2 years. It is becoming increasingly commonplace for a newly diagnosed child to be referred to an implant center even prior to the age of 2 to begin the candidacy evaluation which is part of preimplant screening. When this is the case, it is possible that the implant team is the first agency to whom the parents are sent when looking for services for their child. In this case, it is incumbent upon the implant center team to be knowledgeable about the communication and educational options available to children with hearing loss. Choices that parents make at this time may affect choices that will be open to them in the future. Well-meaning professionals in the field of implantation must keep in mind that it is indeed the parents' right to make informed decisions about their child's future. A balanced presentation of the issues involved in communication and education alternatives is the cornerstone for building a trusting partnership with the family of a potential implant candidate. It is beyond the scope of this book to elaborate on the educational and communication issues; therefore, the reader is directed to Schwartz (1987) for more detail.

■❑ THE NEWLY DIAGNOSED CHILD

A newly identified child must immediately register with the appropriate agency in order to be eligible for services. In many states, it is the Department of Education which is responsible for service provision to the birth to 3 year population. In other states, it is the responsibility of the Division of Maternal and Child Health. Regardless of the agency that provides the service, children below the age of 3 are most often enrolled in an early intervention program which provides both home-based and center-based services. Intervention is often aimed at the parent, since it is the parent who is responsible for most of the early learning that occurs during these formative years (Manolson, 1985). In fact the Educational Agency providing the service is mandated by law to write an Individualized Family Service Plan (IFSP). Thus, the needs of the entire family are taken into account when planning intervention, not simply the needs of the child with the hearing loss.

Early intervention programs generally provide counseling or support groups for parents still coping with the fact their child is deaf. They also disseminate information about hearing aids and other assistive devices and help parents establish communication with their child at home. In most cases, there is language enrichment work provided directly to the child. When the child enrolled in an early intervention program is also a candidate for a cochlear implant, there are specific tasks in which the interventionist can engage the child. These can accelerate the candidacy selection process and promote the child's later use of the implant.

■❑ TASKS FOR THE EARLY INTERVENTIONIST OF AN IMPLANT CANDIDATE

Facilitating Language

It is not a coincidence that the most important task for the early interventionist of an implant candidate is also one of the primary responsibilities of early intervention. Beyond audiologic criteria, the most compelling factor in the implantation of the young child is the degree to which he has begun to use a formalized system of language. It does not matter whether the language is oral or signed. The importance is that the child demonstrates an understanding that communication is functional. He must also demonstrate the use of abstract yet conventional symbols (either words or signs) to have needs and wants met and to comment on his environment. Children who demonstrate this ability are likely to make greater use of their implant, having already deciphered the symbolic code of language. Any language curriculum which targets early pragmatic skills and the development of single words across semantic categories is likely to be appropriate for the prospective implant candidate.

Teaching the Stimulus-Response Paradigm

Young children who can demonstrate an understanding of the stimulus-response paradigm give more reliable results on hearing tests and can be more active participants in the postimplant tuning of the speech processor. Asking a toddler to *wait* for a word, a sign, or some sort of action from the teacher/therapist is difficult enough. Asking him to then perform a task or say or sign something in response makes it doubly difficult. Yet, this is a learned behavior which can be taught. The teacher/therapist is encouraged to include activities which develop stimulus-response awareness into direct instruction sessions. Teaching this concept does not need to be linked to listening or language initially. In fact, with very young children, it may be more beneficial to teach the concept through large motor activities. Designing a task so that a child is directed to run when the teacher waves a flag is one way to teach the paradigm. In another task, the child can open a box when the teacher claps her hands. The task itself is not important as long as the child is learning to wait for the teacher before responding. Success in gross motor activities can then be used as the foundation for shaping the response in other visual and linguistic tasks.

Communicating That Sound Carries Meaning

For the very young child who has never heard, it is important to attempt to communicate that sound has meaning. The teacher/therapist should use language that describes sound and should acknowledge the role that it plays in our environment. For example, if the teacher/therapist is working with the child in a room and someone comes to the door and knocks, she should indicate to the child that a sound has been made which signals to her that someone is outside the door. This communicates to the child that the sound of knocking can be heard and alerts the person *inside* that someone is *outside* and wants to come in. One early intervention program used this strategy in the group classroom repeatedly; anytime the teacher or the aide left the room she would knock on the door of the classroom on returning. The teacher inside the classroom would call attention to the knocking and ask the children to listen. She would then instruct one of the children to call out, "Come in!"

Encouraging the Use of a Full Voice by Parents When Signing

To optimize the benefits of the cochlear implant, parents need to speak in a sufficiently but comfortably loud voice so that the child can listen. In some cases, parents of children enrolled in total communication programs sign to their child with a whispered voice or with no voice at all. This does not often represent a conscious decision, but rather a habit that develops. When parents first begin to sign they may feel awkward and slow. Signing and talking at the same time may be laborious and may make their speech sound unnatural. Parents may eliminate the spoken aspect of their message to focus on the sign. Additionally parents may not talk because the child has shown no responsiveness to speech. The attitude of "he can't hear me anyway" may develop and the habit of signing without voice may be firmly entrenched. It is recommended that all interventionists with parents who have chosen the total communication option monitor simultaneous communication closely.

Encouraging Natural and Easy Vocalizations

We know that hearing helps us monitor voice production and that there is a direct relationship between degree of hearing loss and voice quality (Boothroyd, 1982). Because the child who is an implant candidate gets limited, if any, auditory feedback from his hearing aids, he relies on kinesthetic feedback for voice production. The well intentioned speech-language pathologist or classroom teacher who uses tactile cues (such as a hand on the throat) may be inadvertently encouraging tensing of the vocal folds. This may produce a harsh or strident voice. If vocalizations are forced or cued by tactile strategies, an unnatural voice quality may develop. One of the outcomes of implantation is the child's ability to hear his own voice for the purpose of monitoring speech production. Thus, the potential for developing a natural sounding voice is attainable after implantation. However, if a harsh quality is developed prior to implantation, improving quality may be a necessary and difficult step in developing overall intelligibility of speech. Thus, encouraging a child to "talk" (either alone or while signing) might be a better prompt than "use your voice," for it deemphasizes the attention to the laryngeal area. If, prior to implantation, establishing the concept of voicing is difficult, a child may be encouraged to feel the resonance of voicing in the chest area.

Laying the proper foundation during the period of candidacy selection with very young children supports the entry into the postimplant phase. Many of the tasks begun during the candidacy phase are continued after the child receives the device. Parents who are frustrated by the lack of auditory responsiveness of their child may abandon much of this early work. These parents may believe that the cochlear implant will provide the auditory information necessary and that practice with conventional hearing aids is not productive. They lack the understanding that exposure to these activities at early stages will ease the transition once the child is implanted.

■ THE NEWLY IMPLANTED 2-YEAR-OLD

Perhaps the most significant difference between a 2-year-old implant user and a child who is newly implanted but older is the potential for wearing issues to occur. Oftentimes, the 3- and 4-year-old is a much more compliant child when wearing the implant throughout the day. Some 2-year-olds, however, will add wearing the device to their list of situations to battle with their parents. If the child is difficult to manage in everyday routines, it is likely that wearing the device may be problematic as well. It is important to provide assistance to the parents at this time. The frustration of coaxing the child to wear the device is often exacerbated by the parents' feelings of pressure for validation of their decision to implant. If a willful child sees that wearing the device is yet another opportunity for him to exert control over his parents, he may simply refuse to put it on. In some cases, after a battle, the child may acquiesce for a short time and then remove the microphone and transmitter coil and allow it to dangle. (One must be careful not to interpret the accidental dislodging of the headpiece with a willful act by the controlling child. The cords of the headpiece may be snagged, which results in the headset falling. The young child will be unable to replace it without assistance from a parent or teacher.)

Implant center staff may work cooperatively with the early interventionist to address wearing problems. In some instances, a simple approach that rewards wear time may be all that is necessary. Giving the child stickers for putting the device on may be helpful.

In other cases, parents may have larger issues of management and control which need to be addressed. In these instances, a comprehensive plan to provide support and guidance to the parents in child management may need to be developed. The use of negative reinforcers may be the best solution to battle-weary parents who are struggling to maintain control. In a strategy called *planned ignoring,* parents do not get upset if the child refuses to wear the device; nor do they insist that the child put it on. Parents are instructed to offer the device to the child. If the child refuses, they are to indicate that without the device there will be no activity or interaction. At regular intervals, they are to offer the child the device and indicate which activities the child will be missing because of the lack of cooperation. For children who have been used to causing a scene over this issue, this turnabout is extremely puzzling. However, its power is in the dramatic change in the parental coping strategy. Giving parents permission to avoid struggling with the child to wear the device may be the better short-term solution for all involved.

■□ DESIGNING POSTIMPLANT HABILITATION

The young implant recipient's postimplant habilitation must follow developmental milestones in the areas of language and audition. It cannot be overstated that continued linguistic development is the cornerstone of auditory habilitation. All too often, children with the implant reach an auditory ceiling because of linguistic limitations. That is, they appear to have reached the limit of their auditory ability when, in fact, it is difficulty with the language of a particular activity which creates an artificial cap on their auditory skills. However, this ceiling is real enough functionally because no further progress can be made unless further language development is accomplished. The teacher/therapist now has an added tool to assist in the task of language development—a sensation of hearing. Finding ways to develop language while at the same time maximizing the potential of the device is the primary objective of the teacher/therapist.

Auditory Learning Revisited

The concept of auditory learning was introduced in Chapter 7, and its practical application for the young implant recipient will be explored here. Recall that auditory learning emphasizes the relationship between listening and the child's speech and spoken language level, his cognitive or intellectual ability, and his everyday life experiences. As such, auditory learning should be compatible with the existing curriculum of most early intervention and preschool programs which value audition as a component of their comprehensive educational plan.

Incorporating Listening Activities Into the Existing Preschool Curriculum

To gain the support of the classroom teacher and the school-based speech/language pathologist, it is necessary to demonstrate some familiarity with the demands and the realities of the school day. The educational consultant model supported in this text requires on-site observation by the implant center educator so that specific recommendations about how to incorporate listening into the classroom can be made. After spending time in the classroom and becoming familiar with the particular classroom's routines, the educational consultant can use real-life examples for maximizing listening opportunities. Because many of the young children are working at the very early level of listening (e.g., detection of sound or identification of patterns), opportunities to provide listening practice for these skills in meaningful contexts are brought to the teacher's attention. The teacher is encouraged to take an extra moment when names are called for lining up for gym, taking a turn at the calendar, or getting the lunchboxes from the cubby, to make these listening-only tasks.

The heart of any preschool classroom, however, is the unit or theme that the teacher plans as the basis of her daily activities. While some units can last as long as a month, such as the Community Helper Unit or Theme, many weekly units may revolve around the reading of a children's book. Oftentimes art, language, science, or social studies and even snack activities are related to the reading. The creative teacher should be encouraged to develop some auditory lessons which also relate to the story reading or other unit theme.

■ A UNIT-BASED APPROACH TO DEVELOPING AUDITORY SKILLS

One popular children's book which seems to lend itself easily to a theme or unit approach is the story of *The Very Hungry Caterpillar* by Eric Carle (1969). This delightful story tells of the brief life of a caterpillar from the time he pops out of his egg to his transformation into a beautiful butterfly. We follow the caterpillar as he eats his way through the days of the week: healthy fruit snacks for the weekdays and a strange assortment of foods on Saturday that includes swiss cheese, a slice of salami, and a piece of chocolate cake. The colorful illustrations, the repetitious refrain found in the text, and the "surprise ending" make it a favorite story for the preschool set. Teachers across the country introduce this story to their class and provide a host of follow-up activities which reinforce and expand on the text.

Heading the list of recommended follow-up activities is the recreation of the story with a caterpillar puppet and cardboard food cutouts. The teacher can produce a large plastic bag that can become the caterpillar's cocoon and the place where the caterpillar hand puppet changes into a tissue paper butterfly. Art activities that create very hungry caterpillars with egg cartons and pipe cleaners or craft shop pom-poms may be appropriate, as would snack activities that allow the children to eat the same fruits as the very hungry caterpillar. Because the caterpillar eats increasing numbers of fruit on successive days of the week, math activities may also be included. Although numerals do not appear in the text, matching sets with one to five items to the numeral (or number word) is appropriate. Because the numeral words one through five actually appear in the text, matching print to the numerals is another reinforcing activity in math and reading. In science, teaching the life cycle of the caterpillar or comparing the caterpillar to other insects are also lessons related to *The Very Hungry Caterpillar* theme.

Designing additional activities which are auditory in nature can also be simple if the teacher or therapist has a protocol to follow. Once the steps of the protocol are identified, they can be adapted for use with any story or unit that the teacher/therapist plans for the class. The six steps outlined in the protocol in Figure 8–1 encourage the teacher to choose vocabulary and language from the story and use these as the basis for designing auditory tasks.

When the protocol is applied to the story of *The Very Hungry Caterpillar* and the first and second tasks have been combined the vocabulary list displayed in Figure 8–2 results.

Protocol for designing auditory lessons to accompany a classroom unit.

1. Identify key vocabulary used within the unit.

2. Categorize the vocabulary into one syllable, two syllable, or polysyllabic lists.

3. Briefly analyze the acoustic information available in the vocabulary lists.

4. Rewrite the story or unit into a brief paragraph recalling the major points or the key concepts. Be sure that sentences vary in length and/or pattern.

5. Identify the auditory skill level of the children in the class.

6. Design appropriate listening activities that reflect the child's linguistic abilities as well.

Figure 8–1
Protocol for designing auditory lessons.

Vocabulary Categorization

ONE SYLLABLE	TWO SYLLABLES	MULTISYLLABIC
leaf	apple	caterpillar
plums	pickle	strawberries
cheese	sausage	oranges
pears	cupcake	chocolate cake
		ice cream cone
		salami
		lollipop
		cherry pie
		watermelon

****

	cocoon	butterfly

****

one	Sunday	Saturday
two	Monday	
three	Tuesday	
four	Wednesday	
five	Thursday	
	Friday	

Figure 8–2
The Very Hungry Caterpillar vocabulary categories.

A quick and simple analysis of the key vocabulary words reveals that there are a large number of multisyllabic words or word combinations which represent food items eaten by the caterpillar. This suggests that pattern recognition can be easily practiced by comparing the multisyllabic words to the single syllable words. The analysis also reveals that all of the number words and most of the days of the week words have similar syllable length—one syllable for number words and two syllables for the day words. This suggests that making listening comparisons within the content category of numbers, for example, would only be appropriate for children who demonstrate some ability to process segmental information. That is, because the *word patterns* are all the same, children must be able to hear differences in the vowels of the number words in order to discriminate or identify them. The same holds true for the days of the week words; in fact, because all of the day words have the same second syllable (day) children asked to discriminate between these words will have to do so on the basis of the auditory information presented in the first syllable (e.g., Sun, Mon, Tooz, Wenz, Thurs, Fry).

The next step of the protocol suggests that a short paragraph summarizing the key points of the story be written. The recreated text appears in the form of a chart or language experience story complete with simple illustrations that help the children "read" the text (see Figure 8–3).

The sentences in this retelling of *The Very Hungry Caterpillar* have been written purposefully, ensuring that the length and patterns of the sentences vary. In this way, the story sentences can easily be used in tasks of pattern perception. Note that in the first sentence (POP! The caterpillar came out of the egg) the use of the exclamation as the introductory word makes that sentence quite different in pattern from the others. Specific attention to patterns is also evident in sentence three. In this sentence, the use of seriation, (pears, apples, plums, and a cupcake) creates still another pattern. Sentences four, five, and seven (He felt sick because he ate so much food; After he ate a leaf, he felt better; and He became a beautiful butterfly) all have the same number of total syllables. The patterns of the sentences vary enough so that it is likely that a child could differentiate among them by relying only on pattern information.

The next step in the protocol suggests that the teacher/therapist identify the auditory skills of the children in her class so that she may design effective listening activities. Some auditory skills which may be appropriate for implant users include tasks of pattern perception, closed set word identification, open set word identification, and tasks

The Very Hungry Caterpillar

POP! the caterpillar came out of the egg.

He started to look for some food.

He ate pears, apples, plums and a cupcake.

He felt sick because he ate so much food.

After he ate a leaf, he felt better.

The caterpillar made a cocoon and went to sleep.

He became a beautiful butterfly.

Figure 8–3
The Very Hungry Caterpillar experience story.

of auditory comprehension. Recall that each of these auditory skills should be practiced at a number of language levels so that a skill is not simply developed in a single linguistic context. The final step in the protocol dictates the actual design of the tasks. Activities must be generated with the knowledge of the child's linguistic abilities reflected in the level of the stimuli. The following seven activities are provided as examples of tasks appropriate for children of differing abilities. It is not intended as a sequence of activities through which to take a single child. However, this should become obvious as the activities are outlined requiring a range of skill levels.

Activity 1

Skill: Pattern perception

Language level of stimulus: Single word in isolation

Task: Identify the target word "caterpillar" presented randomly in a list of other one syllable words

Materials: Toy caterpillar and a gameboard with a path from start to finish

Procedure: Teacher develops stimulus list from story vocabulary. Pictures of these words are put on index cards. One multisyllabic word is selected as the target word; multiple pictures of the target word are made and shuffled into the "deck." Words are presented one at a time. When the child hears the target word, he responds by approximating the target word. If he does not hear the target word he makes no response. If correct, he is reinforced by making his egg carton caterpillar walk across a gameboard. After looking and listening trials and auditory only practice, the task is reversed. The child shuffles the deck and produces the stimulus words as prompted by the pictures. The teacher listens for contrasts in multisyllabic word and single word production

Sample dialog:

Teacher: We have been talking all week about caterpillars. This is a very important word in our story. It is a long word with many sounds in it. Listen to the word (Teacher says slowly): CAT ER PIL ER. That has many sounds. We will play a listening game now with that word. I will say some words. They are all story words. I might say caterpillar, our special story word, or I might say plum. Plum is a word in the story too. It is short. It only has one sound. It is not the special word. You will have to listen for our special story word. When you hear the special story word, caterpillar, tell me yes. If you do not hear the word tell me no. When you are correct, you can move the caterpillar across the table. First, we will try it with looking and listening. Then we try it with listening only.

(continued)

Teacher:	(reading from cards) CHEESE
Child:	no
Teacher:	PLUMS
Child:	no
Teacher:	CATERPILLAR
Child:	yes
Teacher:	(acknowledges correct answer and reinforces) Now, let's try it with listening only. (still reading from cards but her mouth is no longer visible) CATERPILLAR
Child:	yes
Teacher:	PEARS
Child:	no
Teacher:	CHEESE
Child:	no
Teacher:	CATERPILLAR
Child:	yes

After each correct response, the child is allowed to move his egg carton caterpillar across the gameboard. "Play" continues until the child reaches the finish line. At this point the teacher can offer the child a turn "to be the teacher." Now, the task becomes a productive one. When prompted by the appropriate picture card, the child must produce some approximation of the multisyllable word, caterpillar, so that it is distinguishable from the one syllable words in the list. The teacher may want to make a decision about how she will respond to speech productions that are in error. That is, the word caterpillar may be said by the child with less that the required four syllables (e.g., A ER PI). Depending on the child's abilities, this may be accepted as his best attempt, or the teacher may prompt for an approximation of the vowel in the final syllable. Regardless, it is recommended that the teacher refrain from attempting to correct articulation; the point of this portion of the activity is to produce syllables, not particular consonants.

Working with Error Responses

In the listening example above, the child did not make any errors. It is likely that this auditory task will be easy if the child responds appropriately when the task is presented with audition and vision together. If, however, the child does make mistakes (responding when a one syllable word is given, or failing to respond when the target word is presented) the teacher should indicate to the child that the stimulus presented required a different response. The teacher tells the child the stimulus word and reinforces the appropriate response. The dialog for this exchange might sound like this:

Teacher:	(presents LEAF)
Child:	yes
Teacher:	(with mouth uncovered and adding signs, if necessary) I didn't say CATERPILLAR, I said LEAF. Listen to the difference (Teacher points to the stimulus pictures as she says the words) CATERPILLAR-LEAF; CATERPILLAR-LEAF. Listen again, I will say LEAF. (Teacher covers mouth) LEAF
Child:	no
Teacher:	Now listen again. PEARS
Child:	no

Similarly, if the teacher presents the target word and the child fails to respond, the teacher should indicate to the child that the target word has been said. She tells the child that the appropriate response is yes, because the target word has been produced. She gives the child multiple opportunities to listen to the target word for practice and then resumes the random presentation of the target in the one syllable list. Dialog representing this exchange appears below.

Teacher:	(presents CATERPILLAR)
Child:	no
Teacher:	(with mouth uncovered and adding signs, if necessary) I said CATERPILLAR this time. Listen again while I say caterpillar. CATERPILLAR. You say it.
Child:	(approximates caterpillar)
Teacher:	Listen one more time to caterpillar. CATER-PILLAR. OK. Now let's try again (Teacher continues as above).

In the following activity, the skill continues to be pattern perception. The language level of the stimulus remains at the single word level. Because these targets are words in isolation, there is a low level of linguistic complexity in this task. The difference between this activity and the first is that the child must now identify which one of two words was said by the teacher based on pattern perception.

Activity 2

Skill: Pattern perception

Language level of stimulus: Single word in isolation

Task: Choose from two alternatives the single or polysyllabic word that is said by the teacher

Materials: Small pieces of plastic fruit to serve as markers for responses

Procedure: Using the picture cards as recommended for development in activity one, the teacher reviews all single syllable and multisyllable vocabulary words. She then takes a one syllable word picture card and a multisyllable word picture card and places them on the table in front of the child. The child is asked to label the items pictured. In a looking and listening trial, the teacher presents one of the words, and the child identifies which word he heard by repeating the stimulus. He also marks his response by

(continued)

placing a miniature strawberry in front of the picture named. The teacher may provide multiple trials with the same set or continually make changing sets. As indicated in Activity 1, the teacher reverses roles and allows the child to present the stimuli.

Sample dialog:

Teacher: Here are some picture cards of words from our story. Let's review all the words that are important to the story. (Child identifies pictures; Teacher helps with the production of the proper number of syllables.) Here are two pictures from the story. This is a LOLLIPOP and this is CHEESE. One word is long and one word is short. I will say one of the words. Maybe I will say LOLLIPOP or maybe I will say CHEESE. You will tell me which one I said. You can put a little strawberry in front of the picture that I say. First, we will try it with looking and listening. Then we try it with listening only.

Teacher: CHEESE

Child: (repeats cheese and puts a strawberry in front of the picture) (Multiple looking and listening trials will likely be necessary. Only a single trial is presented here for illustration purposes.)

Teacher: That's correct. Now try with listening only. CHEESE

Child: (repeats cheese and puts a strawberry in front of the picture)

Teacher: Good. LOLLIPOP

Child: (repeats lollipop and puts a strawberry in front of the picture)

Teacher: CHEESE

Child: (says lollipop)

(continued)

Teacher:	(stops the child from putting the strawberry in front of the wrong picture) I said CHEESE. That is the short word. Listen again. CHEESE. OK, now we will try again. LOLLIPOP
Child:	(says lollipop)
Teacher:	(continues to randomly present either the stimuli CHEESE or LOLLIPOP. When the miniature strawberries have been used up, teacher can reverse roles and the child produces the stimuli. The teacher checks to see if the child can make a difference productively between a single syllable and a multisyllable word.)

In the third recommended activity, the child is still asked to listen to the patterns of words. In this activity the teacher changes the complexity of the linguistic environment. Now, the demands of the task are greater because the target word appears at the end of a short sentence. The child must filter past the other words in the sentence and listen for the one word that is different between the two sentences.

Activity 3

Skill: Pattern perception

Language level of stimulus: Single word in a sentence context

Task: Perform a task as prompted by a stimulus sentence

Materials: Caterpillar puppet and food miniatures or pictures of food items

Procedure: Using the carrier phrases "the caterpillar wants a _____" or "the caterpillar wants some_____" the teacher will fill in the blank with a food word that is either a single syllable or a multisyllabic word. The

(continued)

teacher sets up the task with a two-item choice (one a single syllable word and one a multisyllable word) in a looking and listening trial. The teacher says a sentence and the child "feeds" a caterpillar puppet with the appropriate miniature or picture of the food named. When the child demonstrates success with the looking and listening task, the teacher moves to auditory only production. Turns at giving directions and feeding the caterpillar are alternated

Sample dialog:

Teacher:	Here is our caterpillar puppet from our story. He is a very hungry caterpillar today. We will feed him some of his favorite foods. We have a pear, a plum, some cheese, a leaf, a strawberry, some chocolate cake, some salami, a lollipop, some cherry pie, and some watermelon. I will tell you what the caterpillar wants and you can feed it to him. Maybe he'll want a plum or maybe he'll want a strawberry. Let's try one. (The teacher can, depending on the age and motivation of the child, pretend that the caterpillar puppet tells her what he wants.)
Teacher:	THE CATERPILLAR WANTS A STRAW-BERRY.
Child:	(feeds the caterpillar puppet the strawberry)
Teacher:	THE CATERPILLAR WANTS A PLUM.
Child:	(feeds the caterpillar the plum)
Teacher:	OK Let's try with listening only. Maybe the caterpillar will want some chocolate cake or maybe he will want some cheese. (Note that in these choices the teacher selects foods that require the same quantifying adjective so that the carrier phrase would be exactly the same for both choices—The

(continued)

	caterpillar wants some _____. If the choices were: "The caterpillar wants some chocolate cake" and "The caterpillar wants a leaf," the carrier phrase would be different—"The caterpillar wants *some* . . ." and "The caterpillar wants *a* . . .") THE CATERPILLAR WANTS SOME CHOCOLATE CAKE.
Child:	(feeds the caterpillar chocolate cake)
Teacher:	That's correct! Now listen again. Maybe he will want a STRAWBERRY or maybe he will want a LEAF. Ready. THE CATERPILLAR WANTS A LEAF.
Child:	(responds by feeding the caterpillar a leaf)
Teacher:	Now, maybe he will want some salami or some cheese. THE CATERPILLAR WANTS SOME CHEESE.
Child:	(responds by feeding the caterpillar some cheese)

As in other activities, the child is given a number of listening trials either in straight turns or in alternating turns with the teacher. It will be necessary for the child to make an attempt at producing speech that is intelligible enough to make a differentiation between sentences. Even if the child has difficulty in producing an entire intelligible sentence, he must understand that his best effort must come at producing speech that will help the teacher tell the difference between the two targets. Implementing the concept of engineering the linguistic environment, the teacher can alter the carrier phrase to change the location of the auditory target. The same task can be presented for additional practice by asking the child to listen to this carrier "I want a/some _____," said the caterpillar.

In Activity 4, the auditory skill remains at the level of pattern perception, but now sentences are used as the stimuli. This activity should also be presented to children who are successful with Activity 3; it represents movement along the language continuum with the auditory skill of pattern perception.

Activity 4

Skill: Pattern perception

Language level of stimulus: Sentences

Task: Identify the sentence read by the teacher

Materials: Teacher-made experience story of the very hungry caterpillar

Procedure: Teacher reviews all sentences on the chart with the child. She selects two sentences to contrast and asks the child to listen to the one that she says. The child identifies the sentence by pointing to it on the chart and "reading" it back to the rest of the class.

Sample dialog:

Teacher:	Today we will be looking at our story chart that we wrote about the Very Hungry Caterpillar. We will be using the chart to practice listening. I will point to two sentences and then I will say one of the sentences. You point to the sentence that I say and then read it to the rest of the class. Let's try one with looking and listening. Maybe I will say HE ATE PEARS, APPLES, PLUMS, AND A CUPCAKE or HE BECAME A BEAUTIFUL BUTTERFLY. Ready. HE BECAME A BEAUTIFUL BUTTERFLY.
Child:	(points to the correct sentence and reads it aloud)
Teacher:	OK. Let's try with listening only. The two sentences that you need to listen for are: POP! THE CATERPILLAR CAME OUT OF THE EGG and AFTER HE ATE A LEAF, HE FELT BETTER. Ready. AFTER HE ATE A LEAF HE FELT BETTER.
Child:	(points to the correct sentence on the chart and reads it)

When a child is successful with this task, the set can be enlarged to include more and more sentences until the entire chart becomes a closed set of choices. This must be done slowly, however, so that the child does not experience frustration or failure. The teacher must always respond to errors by making the task more simplistic so that the child can be successful. When newly implanted children are successful with tasks of pattern perception and move into closed and open set tasks, modification to chart story activities tap more advanced auditory skills. See the discussion in Chapter 9 on this issue.

Activity 5 outlines a task dependent on the skill of closed set word identification. This is accomplished using segmental information rather than pattern information. It represents a significant advancement in auditory skill ability.

Activity 5

Skill: Closed set word identification

Language level of stimulus: Single words

Task: Select the target word from a set of four words using segmental cues

Materials: Picture cards of vocabulary items

Procedure: Teacher reviews all vocabulary words from the polysyllabic list. She chooses four word cards and places them on the table in front of the child. She reviews the items in the set and presents one word auditorally. The child responds by turning the card over and repeating the word.

Sample dialog:

Teacher: For our listening practice today we will be working with some words from *The Very Hungry Caterpillar* story. These are the words we will be using: caterpillar, strawberries, oranges, chocolate cake, ice cream cone, salami, lollipop, cherry pie, and watermelon. I will choose four words to listen to, and you will need to pick the word that I say. Let's practice first with looking and listening. The four choices are oranges, salami, lollipop, and cherry pie. Ready. ORANGES.

Child: (points to the word oranges)

Teacher: OK. Turn it over and say the word yourself.

(continued)

Child:	oranges
Teacher:	Good. (She removes the word card and replaces it with another keeping the set at four). Let's try with listening only now. Ready. LOLLIPOP.
Child:	(turns the lollipop card over and says the word)
Teacher:	Good. (She removes the identified card replaces it with another and continues the trials.)

As indicated above, one way to increase the complexity of this task is to enlarge the closed set. A second option is to move the targets from multisyllabic words to two syllable words (as in most of the days of the week). A third task requires creating a closed set of one syllable words. This is the most difficult of the closed set word identification tasks because the auditory information is so brief that there is less chance of getting pieces of information to help the child figure out the target word.

Increasing the linguistic complexity of the task while at the same time targeting word identification can be yet another variation in the unit plan. One way in this can be accomplished is to reformat the feeding the caterpillar task described in Activity 3. Although the activity remains the same, the stimuli become closed sets of polysyllabic or single syllable words imbedded in the carriers: "The caterpillar wants _____ (watermelon, salami, strawberries, chocolate cake)," or "I want_____," said the caterpillar (cheese, plums, pears, leaves).

Demonstrating the skill of open set word identification is one that generally takes a significant amount of practice listening with the implant. It is presented here for illustrative purposes; there may be some children who can perform this task. It is likely, however, that this ability may not be demonstrated by children who are among the newly implanted. Open set word identification represents a milestone accomplishment in listening and is not achieved by all children with implants. (Chapter 11 details performance expectations in greater detail.) Activity 6 is offered with this caveat and further serves to illustrate the concept that any auditory skill can be practiced using this format.

The teacher continues to present fruit names without regard to syllable length—the only constraint being the limitations of the child's

Activity 6

Skill: Open set word identification

Language level of stimulus: Single word in isolation

Task: Identify a fruit word as either being one mentioned in the story or not mentioned in the story

Materials: None

Procedure: Selecting a category such as fruit, the teacher presents names of fruits auditorially and the child is asked to respond whether or not the item named is a vocabulary word from the story or not from the story.

Sample dialog:

Teacher:	The Very Hungry Caterpillar ate a lot of different things in the story. One of the healthy foods he ate was fruit. Can you think of some of the fruit that he ate?
Child:	strawberries and plums
Teacher:	Yes, he ate both of those fruits. Can you think of a fruit that you like to eat that was not in the story?
Child:	He didn't eat banana.
Teacher:	That's right. He didn't eat any bananas. Let's try a listening game about the Very Hungry Caterpillar and the fruit that he ate. I'll say the name of a fruit. You tell me if it was a fruit in the story or not in the story. Let's try a few before we try with listening only. Ready. PLUM.
Child:	In the story.
Teacher:	Correct. The caterpillar ate a plum. How about another one? LEMON.
Child:	That not in the story.
Teacher:	Yes, good. You have the idea. Now we'll try with listening only.

own vocabulary. Thus, the teacher would be wise to refrain, perhaps, from the names of less familiar, exotic fruit such as kiwi or mango. Increases in the language demands of the task by changing the linguistic environment of the stimulus should be made if, and only if, the child has consistent success with the task as presented. If he has, the adapted task presents the target in a sentence context, "Did the caterpillar eat a lime?"

Another variation on this task is to refrain from specifying the food category as was done in the Activity 6. This increases the possibilities of target words that the child is asked to judge: for example, Did the caterpillar eat a hamburger? a strawberry? a candy cane? Finally, the teacher may devise a task in which the child is asked to recognize sentences from the Very Hungry Caterpillar chart versus those from another story chart. For sophisticated listeners, the teacher could present sentences from a number of different stories and the child's task is to name the story that a particular "famous line" is from.

The final activity present for the Very Hungry Caterpillar unit addresses phoneme detection. While detecting phonemes may seem to be a basic task, the context is a sophisticated phonological one. In this activity phoneme detection signals singular or plural items and the child makes a judgment based upon the presence or absence of the /s/ or /z/ phoneme. Thus this detection task is somewhat advanced.

Activity 7

Skill: Phoneme detection

Language level of stimulus: Phoneme in a single word context

Task: Identify either the singular or plural form of fruits that were eaten by the very hungry caterpillar

Materials: Pictures of both singular food items or plural food items eaten by the caterpillar

Procedure: The object of this activity is to have the student perceive the presence or absence of the plural, marked either by the phoneme "s" or "z." Production of these contrasts will be required as well.

Note: a cognitive/linguistic precursor to this activity is the child's understanding of the concept of pluralization

(continued)

Sample dialog:

Teacher:	Our listening activity today is about the food that the Very Hungry Caterpillar ate in our story. We know that he ate a plum and some apples and a lollipop. In our activity today we will be listening to find out if he ate one thing or more than one thing. If you hear apple, it means he ate one thing. If you hear appleZ, it means he ate more than one apple. In our picture, we have three apples. If you listen carefully to the food words and hear "s" or "z" at the end of the word you will know that he ate more than one. If you do not hear "s" or "z" it means he ate only one. When you hear APPLEZ, point to the picture of three apples. If you hear apple and do not hear the Z sound at the end, point to one apple. Let's try first with looking and listening. Ready. APPLE. Did the caterpillar eat one apple or three apples?
Child:	one apple
Teacher:	That's correct. You did not hear the "Z" at the end. Let's try another food. Listen to find out if the caterpillar ate one lollipop or three lollipops. Ready. LOLLIPOPS. Which one did I say?
Child:	lollipops.
Teacher:	Good. Does that tell you one or more than one?
Child:	More than one.
Teacher:	Super! Here is another one. This is a picture of a plum. Here are two plums. Ready. PLUMS. Which one did I say?
Child:	Plums, more than one.
Teacher:	Yes, let's try with listening only.

The teacher continues the trials, alternating turns with the student, if desired. Given the child's success with the task, the teacher can increase task difficulty by imbedding the targets in a carrier sentence: "After the caterpillar ate _____, he went to sleep." This sentence is somewhat contrived to ensure placement of the target in the middle rather than at the end of the sentence. In addition, it is probable that there will be some differences between the articles preceding the target (e.g., a lollipop, some lollipops). If the teacher is careful not to overemphasize the article and presents it in the stream of connected speech before the target, it may not make a marked difference in the auditory task.

■□ SUMMARY

The young deaf child who is considered a candidate for implantation will likely present with educational issues which should be addressed by implant center staff. Guiding parents through early intervention is the first step in preparing the child for implantation. Service providers unfamiliar with the process of implantation may look to the implant center for direction with regard to readying the child for the device. Fortunately, much of what the early intervention specialist already does can be customized for the potential implant recipient. Of paramount importance is the establishment of language and speech, with particular attention to the concept that sound carries meaning. Once a child receives an implant, habilitation continues to be driven by language activities. Minor adaptations to the existing preschool curriculum so that it emphasizes audition can be accomplished using the unit protocol. Activities that add listening to unit-related tasks can be easily designed by the creative teacher.

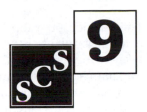

The School-Age Child
with an Implant

The school-age child category spans the time from the beginning of the primary years (age 6) up to and including the preteenage years (age 12). There are two distinct subgroups of implant recipients found within this category. The first is the child who is evaluated and implanted during this period. As knowledge and acceptance of the implant grows, this is a shrinking population. Many parents are now seeking implantation for their children during the early, critical language-learning years. However, there is still a small number of children who, for one reason or another, are candidates during their later elementary school years (age 8 and older). This group may include children with a progressive hearing loss, a late recommendation by hearing health professionals, a diagnosis of Usher syndrome (Chute & Nevins, 1995) or, in some cases, a recommendation from school personnel because of minimal progress using hearing aids alone. The profiles of the candidates in this group are characterized by marked variability; and, despite the fact that the implant serves as a common thread uniting these children, continued marked variability during the postimplant period is likely to be seen.

◼️◻️ IMPLANT VETERANS

The second subgroup in the school age category, is the group who received implants between the ages of 2 and 5 and now have 3 to 6 years of implant use. Although the number of children with 6 years of implant use is still relatively small, this figure will continue to grow, as will the upper end age for years of implant use. At the time when implant veterans enter this school-age phase, they are likely to demonstrate significant auditory abilities not present prior to implantation. New users and implant veterans are two vastly different groups with a range of speech, language, and auditory skills. Nevertheless, making general recommendation for children at this age level is made possible by the implementation of the unit protocol outlined in Chapter 8. The unit theme protocol is appropriate for the school-age child whether the skill level be pattern perception for the newly implanted child or open set speech recognition for the implant veterans. Another key difference between these two groups is the type of school placement in the middle elementary years. It is likely that newly implanted children will be found in self-contained programs for deaf children, while a percentage of the implant veterans may be receiving their education in the mainstream (Nevins & Chute, 1994). The unit protocol may be used in the self-contained classroom and adapted for the mainstream. Before addressing the application of the unit protocol to the school-age child, however, a recommendation for "aggressive auditory management" (Nevins et al., 1991) that capitalizes on the routines of classroom life will be outlined

◼️◻️ CLASSROOM ROUTINES

Good teachers know that establishing routines makes classroom management much easier (Good & Brophy, 1994). Because the concept of routine suggests that an event occurs regularly at a given time, in a given sequence with a fixed "script," it offers the child with an implant an opportunity to use hearing in the activity. For example, if the "getting ready for lunch routine" occurs in the same way every day, the child can make certain predictions about what will happen during the course of that activity. The teacher announces that it is time to clear the desks. Children who have their desks cleared and are sitting quietly, attentive to the teacher, are eligible to have their names called to get their lunchboxes in the first phase of this routine. Once all children have gotten their lunchboxes and have returned to their desks, the next phase of the routine may be lining up to go to the lunchroom. An auditory component can be inserted into each of the phases of this routine by making the name calling activity an auditory-only one. Even children with pattern perception ability are likely to benefit from this real-life auditory practice. Although there may be a few children who cannot participate in this auditory-only activity, there are children with hearing aids who could benefit from this task. The teacher of children with many years of implant use must "up the auditory ante" and make the task more challenging for the implant veterans with greater language and auditory abilities. Rather than simply call a name in an auditory-only mode, the teacher may direct "whoever has on blue jeans" to get their lunchboxes.

■ ROUTINES IN THE MAINSTREAM CLASSROOM

A number of classroom routines appear to be more specific to the mainstream setting. The first, roll call, is found in all school programs and will occur multiple times in schools in which there are classroom changes throughout the day. This activity may be one in which the child must be "coached" into participating and need not be an auditory-only activity initially. The child should be alerted to his place on the roll call list. In fact, he may even be given a written list of names in the order in which they are called. The objective is to become familiar with the stimuli so that after some experience the child's participation is natural and easy. This will enable him to routinely respond "Here!" when his name is called by the teacher.

A second common routine in the mainstream classroom is homework checking. This task especially lends itself to auditory work because there is a predictable sequence to the responses, and the child generally has the answer in front of him. The child with an implant who follows along as answers are read aloud and takes a turn appropriately is demonstrating good in-class listening skills.

■ COORDINATING AUDITORY LEARNING WITH SUPPORT SERVICES

Children must be held auditorally accountable for their participation routine class activities. In some cases, the services of a teacher/interpreter may prevent the child from taking auditory responsibility.

Although it is not the intent to withhold information from a child with interpreter services, it is recommended that he be given the chance to be a full participant in classroom activities. The interpreter may serve as a backup system during routines and must refrain from making the child dependent upon her for all classroom communication. This also holds true for reverse interpreting, that is, voicing for the student when he answers a question. Students should be expected to answer questions directly to the teacher, not to the interpreter. In general, mainstream teachers should be instructed on how to work with a deaf child and with an interpreter in order to prevent "Interpreter Takeover." This phenomenon suggests that classroom exchanges take place between the teacher and the interpreter and not between the teacher and the student. This may happen when the teacher-student relationship is not given a chance to develop because of the fear on the part of the teacher and the interpreter. Consultation from the implant center educator may help mainstream personnel avoid this problem.

■ CAPITALIZING ON CONTENT LESSONS

As was suggested previously in Chapter 8, the elementary school curriculum offers a host of possibilities for the development of auditory lessons that are both educational and meaningful for the child with an implant. Adapting the protocol outlined in the previous chapter for use with content area material is easy. It is not meant to limit the creative teacher in finding new applications of the principles of auditory learning in the classroom. However, it will serve as a starting point for the professional unsure of the task of developing meaningful auditory lessons.

Once again the protocol for designing lessons is presented in Figure 9–1. It may be adapted for use in both the self-contained and mainstreamed classroom; the target material used for illustration purposes at this level is from the science curriculum at approximately a third or fourth grade level. The unit is Weather and our particular topic for demonstrating the application of the protocol is Violent Storms.

The science unit, Weather, and more specifically the topic, Violent Storms, is generally covered in the third or fourth grade curriculum. As part of this topic, students learn the characteristics of four types of violent weather: thunderstorms, tornadoes, hurricanes, and blizzards. Implementing the first and second steps of the protocol simultaneously, the list of categorized vocabulary words that results can be found in Figure 9–2.

Protocol for designing auditory lessons to accompany a classroom unit

1.   Identify key vocabulary used within the unit.

2.   Categorize the vocabulary into one syllable, two syllable, or polysyllabic lists.

3.   Briefly analyze the acoustic information available in the vocabulary lists.

4.   Rewrite the story or a unit topic into a brief paragraph recalling the major points or the key concepts. Be sure that sentences vary in length and/or pattern.

5.   Identify the auditory skill level of the children in the class.

6.   Design appropriate listening activities that reflect the child's linguistic abilities as well as auditory abilities.

Figure 9–1
Protocol for designing auditory lessons.

Weather Vocabulary

clouds	stratus	cumulus
dew	cirrus	water vapor
fog	lightning	evaporate
wind	thunder	tornado
gale	condense	thunderstorm
breeze	droplets	hurricane
gust	funnel	precipitation
		water cycle
		equator

Figure 9–2
Weather vocabulary categories.

A brief analysis of the acoustic features of the vocabulary words found in this unit indicate that, at the single word level, there are seven different vowel sounds in the seven single syllable words listed. This suggests very different acoustic information is available to the child. It further suggests that the closed set task of identifying words based on segmental or vowel information will be easily designed for students at this skill level. The sequence of the activities which follow here are meant to be developmental in nature. Activities 1 through 3 focus on pattern recognition and are outlined for children who are newly implanted during the elementary years. To provide pattern perception practice at the sentence level, the teacher must, according to the protocol, write a brief paragraph recalling the key concepts of the unit. Figure 9–3 outlines the main fact paragraph designed for illustrative purposes on the topic of violent storms. It incorporates both simple and complex language appropriate for a group of deaf children demonstrating some degree of linguistic sophistication.

Although the key concept paragraph is useful for children at this stage of pattern perception, other closed set listening activities can also be developed using the paragraph. Activities 4 and 5, which outline both closed and open set activities, are introduced with the implant veterans in mind. All activities are presented as examples only. The creative teacher will likely be able to develop additional practical activities which serve the dual purpose of reinforcing content and practicing listening skills. The simultaneous presentation of new material and practice of new auditory skills is discouraged. Specific auditory skill work is best accomplished with known or familiar material.

Paragraph of key concepts of the unit

Violent Storms

Violent storms can damage property and injure people.

Hurricanes cause heavy rains and strong winds.

A tornado is a spinning, funnel-shaped cloud.

Storms with thunder and lightning, strong wind and heavy rain are called thunderstorms.

A blizzard is a storm that brings very cold winds and deep snow.

Emergency weather broadcasts help people prepare themselves and their property before a violent storm.

Figure 9–3
"Violent Storms" summary.

Activity 1

Skill: Pattern perception

Language level of stimulus: Single word in isolation

Task: Identify a target three syllable word presented randomly in a list of one syllable words

Materials: Flashcards of one syllable vocabulary words and multiple copies of a three syllable target (e.g., hurricane or tornado or thunderstorm)

Procedure: Using vocabulary list developed for the unit, the teacher reviews vocabulary on flashcards. Additional one syllable words that are familiar to the child and associated with weather may be added to the list to provide more "turns" (e.g., sun, snow, rain). Child listens to and repeats the one syllable stimuli while reading the print on the card. The three syllable word, for example, "hurricane," is presented as the target word. The teacher instructs the child in the procedure—teacher will present a stimulus word and then ask the child "Did you hear "hurricane?" If the child heard the target word he is to respond "Yes, I heard hurricane." If he did not hear the target word he is to respond, "No, I did not hear hurricane." After a looking and listening trial and multiple auditory only trials, the task is reversed. The child shuffles the deck and produces the stimulus words as prompted by the flashcards. The teacher listens for contrasts in multisyllabic and single word production.

Sample Dialog:

Teacher: Because we have been talking about weather and violent storms this week, we will use some of our science vocabulary to help us practice listening. Here are all the words that have one syllable (or sound) in them. Listen as I say the word. Then you say each word after me. (Teacher presents flashcards, saying each word as the child sees the printed word; child repeats each word.) Today we will be listening for the target (special) word "hurricane." It has three syllable (sounds) and is longer

(continued)

than the other words in our list. You will listen to the word that I say and decide if it is our target word "hurricane." I will say the word and then ask you, "Did you hear 'hurricane'?" You will answer, "Yes, I heard 'hurricane'" or "No, I did not hear 'hurricane'." After you listen to all the words, we will trade places and you will say the words and I will answer the questions.

First, we will try it with looking and listening. Then we try it with listening only.

(Teacher picks a card from the face down pile on the desk and gives the child the opportunity to listen and speechread) BREEZE. (Teacher asks the target question) Did you hear hurricane?

Child: I did not hear hurricane

Teacher: Let's try with listening only now. (Teacher presents the next stimulus word while covering her mouth or sitting beside or behind the child so that only auditory cues are available.) SNOW. Did you hear hurricane?

Child: No, I did not hear hurricane.

Presentations by the teacher continue until all cards have been used. If time allows, the child can begin to make presentations of the word on the flashcard. The objective, at this time, is for the child to differentially produce one and three syllable words. As noted in the previous chapter, the teacher may wish to refrain from attempting to correct articulation. The point of this portion of the activity is to produce recognizable syllables not precise consonants. When the task outlined in this activity is difficult for the child and his responses are in error, the teacher should first acknowledge that the response was incorrect. Then, she should provide an auditory and visual presentation of the stimulus that resulted in an error response, followed by an auditory only presentation of the *same* stimulus. In this way, the child is listening to a known stimulus and the trial becomes practice and not a test. (See Chapter 8, Working with Error Responses for additional discussion.)

The following activity continues pattern perception practice. Here the child is asked to identify, based on syllable number, which word was said, given a choice of words that vary in length.

Activity 2

Skill: Pattern perception

Language level of stimulus: Single word in isolation

Task: Choose from two alternatives the single or polysyllabic word that is said by the teacher

Materials: Vocabulary flashcards

Procedure: Using the vocabulary flashcards cards as recommended for development in Activity 1, the teacher reviews all single syllable and multisyllable vocabulary words. Placing a one syllable word card and a multisyllable word card on the table in front of the child, the teacher asks the child to read both cards. After a looking and listening trial, the teacher presents either the multisyllabic or single syllable word in auditory-only trials. The child identifies which word he heard by repeating the stimulus. The teacher may provide multiple trials with the same set or continually make changing sets. After a number of trials, or in alternating turns, the child should also be given the opportunity to present the stimuli.

Sample Dialog:

Teacher: Here are some vocabulary words from our unit on weather. Let's review all the words that are new to our lesson. (Teacher presents flashcard; Child reads vocabulary. Teacher monitors the production of approximations of target words making especially certain that the proper number of syllables is produced.) Let's choose two words to use in our listening practice today. I will choose a one syllable word,

(continued)

	BREEZE, and a three syllable word, TORNADO. Tell me which word I say. First, we will try it with looking and listening. Then we'll try it with listening only.
Teacher:	TORNADO
Child:	(repeats tornado)
Teacher:	That's correct. Listen again. BREEZE
Child:	(repeats breeze)
Teacher:	Good. Let's choose two new words for listening only. Maybe I will say GALE or maybe I will say CUMULUS. Listen. CUMULUS.
Child:	kyum lis
Teacher:	OK, you heard CUMULUS, but listen to the word. It has three syllables, you said only two. You said kyum lis. You need to add a sound: kyum you lis.
Child:	kyum a lis
Teacher:	Better. I heard three sounds.

In this listening trial, the child demonstrates that he can perform the task auditorally. However, his spoken response indicates that the auditory/speech feedback loop may not yet be established or that speech production ability lags behind auditory skill development. This is a phenomenon not uncommon for the newly implanted child. Continued attention to creating a link between listening and talking should help to ameliorate this problem.

In Activity 3, the language level of the stimulus changes from the single word to the sentence. Selection of sentences is made solely on the basis of sentence length and/or patterns.

This exchange points out the importance of *teaching* not just *testing* auditory skills. If the child makes an error response he should be informed of the mistake by the teacher and given the chance to practice the trial again with clues from the teacher (e.g., This sentence is really shorter than the other). If a child makes multiple errors, it is likely that the task is too difficult for him, and greater contrasts need to be

Activity 3

Skill: Pattern perception

Language level of stimulus: Sentences

Task: Identify the sentence read by the teacher

Materials: Teacher developed paragraph listing key concepts of the unit

Procedure: Teacher reviews all sentences in the paragraph with the child. She selects two sentences to contrast and asks the child to listen to the one that she says and repeat it. After a looking and listening trial, the teacher continues to select two sentences but presents only one of the two for the listening trial.

Sample Dialog:

Teacher:	Today for listening practice we will be working with our unit paragraph on violent storms. Let's review the facts we learned about violent storms by reading the sentences in our paragraph. (Children read sentences from the paragraph.) I will read a sentence from the paragraph and you will identify which sentence I read. First, we will try with looking and listening together. You will need to listen for one of these two sentences: A tornado is a spinning, funnel-shaped cloud or Emergency weather broadcasts help people prepare themselves and their property before a violent storm. Ready. A TORNADO IS A SPINNING, FUNNEL-SHAPED CLOUD.
Child:	(points to the correct sentence on the chart and reads it)
Teacher:	OK. Let's try with listening only. The two sentences that you need to listen for this time are: A blizzard is a storm that brings very cold winds and deep snow or

(continued)

	Hurricanes cause heavy rain and strong winds. Ready. HURRICANES CAUSE HEAVY RAIN AND STRONG WINDS.
Child:	A blizzard is a storm that brings very cold winds and deep snow.
Teacher:	No, you chose the wrong sentence. I said this sentence (pointing to the sentence in the paragraph). Listen again as I say this sentence: HURRICANES CAUSE HEAVY RAIN AND STRONG WINDS. Let's try again, listening to these two sentences. Maybe I will say A blizzard is a storm that brings very cold winds and deep snow (as she points to the print) or Hurricanes cause heavy rain and strong winds. This sentence is really shorter than the other sentence. See if you can listen for the difference now. A BLIZZARD IS A STORM THAT BRINGS VERY COLD WIND AND DEEP SNOW.
Child:	A blizzard is a storm that brings very cold winds and deep snow.
Teacher:	Good. That's exactly right!

made in order for him to experience success. Conversely, when the child can easily complete this task, the teacher may wish to "up the cognitive and linguistic ante." By making the response not simply a repetition task, the teacher can encourage "thinking while listening" (Robbins, 1994). Following a Jeopardy-like procedure, the teacher requires the child to make up a question that is appropriate for the fact he has heard. Thus, if the stimulus heard is A BLIZZARD IS A STORM THAT BRINGS VERY COLD WINDS AND DEEP SNOW any of the following questions would be a suitable response:

What does a blizzard bring?

What kind of storm brings deep snow?

What storm brings wind and snow?

What storm brings very cold winds?

Activity 4

Skill: Closed set word identification

Language level of stimulus: Single words

Task: Select the target word from a set of four words using segmental cues

Materials: Vocabulary flashcards

Procedure: Teacher reviews all polysyllabic words from the weather unit list. She chooses four word cards and places them on the desk in front of the child. She names all the items in the set and presents one word in a looking and listening trial. The child responds by choosing the word named and removing the card from the set. The teacher replaces the card with another from the polysyllabic set and presents a stimulus word. Practice continues in this manner until the child has had the opportunity to listen to all the polysyllabic words. The child may then take a turn to present the stimuli and make auditory-only presentations to the teacher.

Alternative responses for a "thinking while listening" task:

- Child chooses the correct answer, turns the card over, and spells the vocabulary word
- Child gives a brief definition of the word
- Child uses the word in a sentence

As a rule of thumb, a child's response to the closed set task should dictate whether the size of the set needs to be increased or decreased. The teacher responds to a child's success by creating increasingly larger sets. Another reaction to success is to shift the listening task from polysyllabic words (in which there is more information available to make judgments) to single syllable contrasts (in which information available is limited to a brief burst). In creating listening sets, the teacher must not ignore the important information provided by an acoustic analysis of the words used in closed set tasks. For example, it would be easier to tell the difference between the single syllable words "gust" and "dew" than between the words "rain" and "gale." In the former example, both consonant and vowels vary; in the latter example, both words have the "long a" sound.

Whenever possible, it is desirable to practice closed set word identification in a sentence context as well as in isolation. "Closed set word identification" presented in isolation is a different task from one in which those same words are embedded in carrier sentences which are exactly the same except for the stimulus item. Depending on the content, designing these tasks may be more or less difficult in some units as opposed to others. In this particular unit, one example of a task requiring closed set word identification in a sentence context gives the child a choice from among the following stimuli:

A tornado is a violent storm.

A hurricane is a violent storm.

A thunderstorm is a violent storm.

The statement "A blizzard is a violent storm" would not be a stimulus item in this set because identification could be made on the basis of pattern perception alone. Making the language of the stimuli more complex changes the "linguistic environment" of the stimuli sufficiently to warrant practice at this level. This is a step often overlooked in auditory skill development programs that do not consider this issue.

Activity 5 presents an open set word identification task that encourages auditory comprehension. The child is not asked to repeat what he has heard as the stimulus, but rather make a judgment about what was heard. When the task is one of categorization, only a limited number of responses may be appropriate.

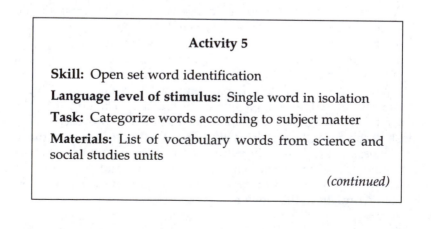

Activity 5

Skill: Open set word identification

Language level of stimulus: Single word in isolation

Task: Categorize words according to subject matter

Materials: List of vocabulary words from science and social studies units

(continued)

Procedure: The teacher instructs the child with regard to the open set categories of vocabulary she will present, for example, words from social studies and words from science. The teacher randomly presents familiar words to the student whose task it is to identify the word as either a science word or a social studies word.

Alternate tasks: Teacher reads character lines from a familiar story and the student names the character that says the line.

- Teacher says the name of a state and the student names the capital city (and vice versa)

- Teacher names examples of matter and the child categorizes it as a solid, liquid, or gas

---

In each of these examples given, the teacher will likely need to probe for the stimulus to which the child believes he is responding, especially when there is a high degree of chance involved in the choices (e.g., a 50–50 chance in categorizing a word as a science or social studies vocabulary word.) This is especially important when the child makes an error response. For the teacher to react appropriately to the incorrect answer and guide the child to an analysis of his error, she will have to ascertain what the child believed he heard.

◼◻ SUMMARY

School-age children, either as new implant users or implant veterans, may benefit from auditory activities which capitalize on the routines of the classroom or the content of the curriculum. Content-based activities must be specifically designed so that they consider the child's auditory *and* language ability. Tasks must be developed which sufficiently challenge the child auditorally while, at the same time, do not frustrate him linguistically. As soon as the child is capable, he should be encouraged to participate in activities which represent the highest level auditory skill—auditory comprehension.

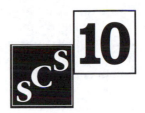

Rehabilitation Strategies for the Adolescent Implant User

Adolescence is probably one of the most difficult times for most individuals. They are not quite children nor are they adults. A day can be completely spoiled if a peer member makes a remark about a piece of clothing, or it can be terrific if the right boy or girl glances their way. It is a time for questioning all types of authority as well as oneself in order to determine one's position in life. For children with profound hearing losses, these same problems exist, often in greater magnitude, because their own ability to communicate with a majority of the population is seriously compromised. The promise of potential hearing benefit from a cochlear implant often leads to misunderstanding by most adolescents and their parents.

At first glance, adolescents represented a group which was initially the most appealing for implantation. These children were already grown and had developed language skills. Erroneously, it was thought that they should have been able to adjust to the new sounds from the cochlear implant with relative ease and speed. Unfortunately, and to the contrary, this group of implant users shows minimal gains even after 2–3 years of implant use. (For performance trends see Chapter 11.) They also demonstrate the highest percentage of nonuse. Assessing this population is almost an art form unto itself, because great pains need to be taken to view the individual as a teenager first and a deaf teenager second. Implant programs that do not have an appreciation for this group's identity will more than likely set themselves up for a disappointment when the adolescent rebellion focuses on the implant. Issues facing the teenager with respect to the candidacy for implantation are addressed in Chapter 4. The purpose of this chapter is to present a format for auditory and speech rehabilitation of this age group in an atmosphere that fosters successful use and avoids boredom.

■❑ AUDITORY AND SPEECH REHABILITATION STRATAGIES

On the average, many teenagers approach their school day with limited excitement and find classroom routines less than appealing. A teacher or a therapist working with an adolescent cannot expect to be greeted with great enthusiasm for an hour of "speech therapy." Does this mean that the rehabilitative process is destined for failure by virtue of the age of the client? Possibly, if the teacher/therapist does not attempt to adjust the therapy so that it maintains interest *and* is effective. Effectiveness of therapy may be quite different for the adolescent implant user compared to the younger child. The majority of children in the adolescent group will have been deaf longer and already subjected to years of therapeutic treatment. That treatment may have been discontinued in the past because minimal progress was demonstrated. Once the adolescent receives the cochlear implant, however, therapy must begin again. This process will be ineffective, if, in assessing the needs of the adolescent, the individual personality traits of the teenager are ignored.

For successful interaction with all adolescents, some evaluation of identity, self-concept, and self-esteem must be obtained. *Identity* develops across a lifespan and is determined by intrapersonal, interpersonal, and environmental variables. *Self-concept* refers to how adolescents view and feel about themselves. *Self-esteem* involves the positive and negative evaluation that results when adolescents evaluate themselves (Knoff, 1987). Often, adolescents with physical and other handicaps have negative body or self-images and have greater difficulty attaining positive self-concepts and self-esteem (Knoff, 1983). These issues become extremely important when addressing both the decision to implant along with the rehabilitative needs of the teenage implant recipient. Ignoring them will lay the groundwork for possible disaster over the course of evaluation and treatment.

The adolescent years are times during which parental goals and children's goals appear to be at opposite ends of the spectrum. In actuality, what parents wish for their child with a disability is similar to what the child himself wishes for—independence, self-direction, and self-support. It is often these goals that initially direct the parents to the implant facility to seek an implant for their teenager. Although these goals are attainable, they do not necessarily require an implant to be realized. Parents who view the implant as being the means to an end and teenagers who view implantation in a similar fashion will be disappointed with the results and approach therapy with a great deal of negative emotion. For the rehabilitative process of implantation to be effective, an approach that assesses the entire child must be undertaken. Deaf adolescents must be evaluated with respect to their ability to cope with their hearing loss. Many of these coping skills can be incorporated into the everyday therapy that is part of the postimplant process.

Traditional auditory training and speech production therapy should include a strong counseling component which addresses the teenager's ability to cope on a day-to-day basis. Teenagers must be able to view their hearing loss as something which may be limiting but not devaluating. Training should include the acquisition of new social and coping skills which may help to restrict the effect of the hearing loss. Deaf teenagers should be taught to value the multitude of other personality traits they possess (e.g., kindness, sportsmanship) and not focus on "normality." This will allow them to recognize their own personality strengths and view the hearing loss as not affecting all aspects of their lives (Spragins, 1987).

Initial Sessions

The best method of determining which coping skills should be emphasized is through direct observation in a natural environment. In most cases, this observation takes place in the classroom, because this is the place the teenager spends a large portion of his day. Analysis of behaviors observed in the classroom may provide valuable information about which communication situations need remediation and which negative habits need to be broken. For example, a profoundly deaf teenager who was reliant on speechreading prior to receiving his implant may have found that the best strategy to avoid errors in understanding was to monopolize the conversation. This is clearly an avoidance reaction to the communication exchange and eventually defeats interaction altogether. Because one of the major benefits of the implant involves the ease with which the user can now speechread, there may be no need to monopolize conversations; speech understanding may now improve. However, if the adolescent has developed some of these negative communication strategies out of habit, he may not realize his new potential in the communication exchange. Remediation in this area cannot begin if the therapist is not aware of the adolescent's pre-rehabilitation behaviors. Oftentimes, the teacher can provide some of the necessary information because she is able to observe the teenager on a daily basis.

When direct observation of particular communication exchanges is not possible, the therapist can role-play communication exchanges with other students. Techniques such as role playing and direct observation will help the therapist better understand the teenager and help establish a trusting relationship. For teachers or therapists who have had no interactive experience with the teenager prior to implantation, there may be a period of adjustment necessary for the teenager to acclimate to speechreading that individual. Therefore, initial sessions with teenage implant users should focus on conversation, information gathering, and the adolescent's discourse style. These sessions can also be employed to determine the special interests, hobbies, and music of the adolescent and should have an informal and relaxed tone. Information gathered at these initial sessions can be useful later in developing listening and speaking activities. Above all, the therapist should use this period to gain the trust and confidence of the adolescent and learn as much as possible about him. From there, the therapy can develop.

Developing Auditory Lessons

There are several approaches which can be used to initiate focused "training" sessions as opposed to information-seeking sessions. Training should begin with the subject (or aspect of sound) that holds the most interest for the teenager. It is often best to begin with half-hour sessions to avoid the possibility of boredom. Oftentimes, teenagers are interested in music and despite their profound hearing losses, spend time watching programs such as MTV. Sessions which deal with listening practice of different musical styles can be fun and teach pattern recognition with material of interest to the student. Beginning sessions should use videos of music that the teenager likes—possibly two or three different songs. As a homework assignment, the adolescent can select several videos which he enjoys and tape them at home. These can be brought to the next session. The therapist should choose among the selected videos to determine if there are any two that are vastly different with respect to pattern perception. The videos should be played with the music and the video presented simultaneously. Once the teenager feels comfortable, the video portion should be removed to determine if the music can be identified based solely on listening. As the skill level increases, and to increase the difficulty of the task, selections in musical style can be made more similar. If the adolescent is willing, the use of other types of music can be introduced. Information from the teenager's music teacher may provide the therapist with material for this type of lesson. For example, if the class is studying opera or classical music, this can be contrasted auditorally with any of the usual rock, rap, or heavy metal songs the teenager might like.

Other subject information from class assignments can be introduced as well. In the example given above, information about the composers being studied in class can be used to bring the student through the different levels of pattern perception, discrimination, and word recognition. The therapist must be on guard, however, to maintain interest. She should be sure to incorporate information about the rock group of interest as well as the class material in use. Material from other classes can be used and interspersed with topics of interest to the adolescent. For example, words, sentences, and concepts from science or history classes can be contrasted with similar types of speech stimuli about cars, clothes, or movies. Once again the key is to maintain interest and a willingness to return and participate. If content material is being used from classroom assignments, the adolescent may begin to notice changes in his understanding of the subject matter because the therapy will act as a review. Better performance in school may also give the teenager more confidence, which will reinforce the therapy overall.

It is extremely important for adolescents to understand that there is a certain amount of responsibility for them in the task. The implant is a tool which can be used to increase auditory awareness. This does not happen on its own. Without significant contribution to the process by the user, results will be poor. Therefore, the therapist should give some form of "homework" to the student. This homework is not the classic type. As noted above, it might consist of bringing videos, music, or favorite magazines to the session. Assigning the traditional types of homework (e.g., drill practice of certain sounds with a parent or partner) will probably be unsuccessful in most cases. However, suggesting to the students that they listen to patterns of music on their favorite CD or cassette may get them started in the right direction.

Developing Speech Production Lessons

Interestingly, speech production is one of the single most important skills in which the adolescent wishes to acquire some improvement. Often, when adolescents are counseled prior to receiving their implant, they are most interested in whether there will be changes in their ability to produce more intelligible speech. Unfortunately, the data available at this time indicate that there is very little change (or at least change that requires years of implant use) with respect to the productive aspects of speech (Parisier & Chute, 1994). Nonetheless, this aspect of rehabilitation should not be ignored.

Once again, by speaking with the adolescent, the therapist can determine those situations in which the teenager might wish to be more intelligible. For example, ordering food in a restaurant may be a circumstance of interest to the teenager. Deaf adolescents often have their parents or a hearing friend order for them. Using role play may help the teenager to cope with these situations better. Mock menus can be generated and the therapist can act as the "waitress." This type of activity incorporates a listening behavior (i.e., when the "waitress" requests the information from the "customer") as well as a productive response. It provides the teenager with an experience with which he is familiar and is able to practice at varying degrees of difficulty and competency.

Practice in the use of the telephone code (Castle, 1988) should also be instituted during training. This code requires some degree of intelligible speech and some amount of auditory perception on the part of the adolescent. It requires that the person using the code be in control of the conversation and be able to explain it to the individual answering the telephone. Auditorally, the telephone code maintains that the user be able to discriminate between the dial tone, telephone signal ring, busy signal, and person responding. In addition, because many people now have answering machines, the listener must be taught to differentiate when the telephone is being answered in person as opposed to a recorded message. After a connection has been made, the hearing-impaired speaker making the call must explain the code to the individual being called. The recipient of the phone call is told that the initiator of the call will ask certain questions. If the answer to the question is "yes" then the recipient is told to say "yes, yes." If the answer to the question is "no" then the recipient should respond "no." If the recipient needs clarification of the questions, she should say "Please repeat" or "I don't understand." In this way, the hearing-impaired adolescent controls the conversation by asking the questions and needs only the ability to discriminate the difference between a one syllable, two syllable, or multisyllable signal. It does, however, require a high degree of speech intelligibility for the precise sentences to be used. These sentences can be practiced both in the individual therapy sessions and at home with a personal tape recorder.

Telephone strategies for use in case of an emergency should be constantly reviewed. Although most deaf teenagers will have access to Telecommunication Devices for the Deaf (TTY), there may be emergency circumstances in which a TTY is unavailable or possibly broken. Providing the adolescent with the ability to respond in cases of emergency fosters independence which is of great importance to most teenagers.

Developing Speechreading Skills

Because one of the major benefits for all users of cochlear implants is the enhancement of *speechreading* skills, this area should be trained and reinforced on a regular basis. The term speechreading is used here to describe input that is both visual and auditory. Materials for speechreading should be chosen by the adolescent. If their interest is in teenager or car magazines, then those stimuli should be used. Forcing the teenager to practice using materials of little or no interest will foster feelings of negativity toward the therapy session. *Speechtracking*, a speechreading technique which requires the individual to repeat verbatim a paragraph which is being read, is probably the best technique to use with this population because it will maintain interest (as long as the materials are chosen carefully), and it provides a speech model that uses continuous discourse (DeFillippo & Scott, 1978).

Speechtracking with the implant activated under good visual conditions will train the teenager in developing or sharpening his speechreading skills. However, the majority of speechreading situations the adolescent may encounter during the day may vary substantially. Therefore, speechreading should be practiced under a variety of visual conditions. For example, distance between the speaker and the speechreader should be varied as should conditions that require speechreading from different angles or with head movement by the speaker. Visual conditions in which the lighting may be less than adequate may also provide the speechreader with a condition that may be similar to that of a dimly lit restaurant. If possible, speechreading in a group where the conversation is shifting from one person to the next is also important to rehearse.

It is often meaningful to query the teenager about speechreading situations which he finds most difficult and attempt to address them. If necessary, the therapy session may need to be relocated if the speechreading problem is related to a specific circumstance. If the speechreading problem stems from a particular teacher, the therapist may need to observe the class to determine the exact nature of the problem. Importantly, input from the adolescent will provide the therapist with information which can help in the construction of therapy sessions.

Postoperative Counseling

Throughout the entire rehabilitative process, an ongoing dialogue should be maintained so that issues of progress, frustration, or disappointment can be addressed immediately. Even the most cooperative and enthusiastic adolescent will sustain periods of depression in which he feels he is no longer making progress. The best method of dealing with these situations is to listen carefully; provide information, explanation, and assurance; and, above all, refrain from minimizing the teenager's feelings. Adolescents need to understand that feeling a particular way is acceptable and that things will change. Fostering as much success as possible during these periods will help bolster the adolescent's self-image and assist him through a critical stage.

Despite every attempt by the speech pathologist or teacher, there are certain adolescents who may need additional counseling from the school psychologist or social worker on a more timely basis. Recommendations for this type of additional help will usually come from the professional or professionals who see the child regularly. At times, counseling may take precedence over formal training for brief intervals to help the teenager get through the more difficult periods. Resumption of therapy after a short moratorium can sometimes be more helpful than continuing therapy when the teenager is unhappy. Flexibility is the key when dealing with this group.

Reward and Reinforcement

Often when therapists deal with younger children, there are a myriad of positive reinforcers which are used throughout and on completion of the session. These rewards may include stickers, food, coloring pictures, puzzles, video games, and verbal praise. This aspect of therapy is often forgotten with the adolescent who is somehow supposed to gain inner satisfaction at his accomplishments on his own. Although verbal praise is given to adolescent clients, this is often not enough for them to feel gratified. Reinforcement mechanisms need to be established by discussing with the teenager those things which might encourage him throughout the process. Sometimes those reinforcements might even include a vacation from therapy. Regardless, it is important to recognize the role of establishing and delivering a reward system that is meaningful to the student.

The Limited User

Despite all the best intentions, counseling, interesting therapy, and positive reinforcers, there are some adolescents who convince themselves early after implantation that the benefits from the device are not worth the hassle of wearing it full time. They may choose instead to wear it only at school and later remove it when they are home or out with friends. They may not wear it at school (especially if they are in a self-contained classroom with manual communication in use) but wear it only when they are out in public. They may wear it only for selected classes or situations. Regardless, they do not use their speech processor on a full-time basis. These "limited users" run the risk of becoming nonusers of the device.

Although there are no guarantees, there are some strategies which can be used to keep the problem in check or to circumvent the problem from developing. Behavioral contracts are sometimes helpful because they require an agreement between the teenager and the parent or teacher with respect to the amount of wear time. These contracts stipulate the exact amount of time or situations in which the device will be worn. In complying with the contract the parents/teachers must agree to avoid questioning the teenager about implant use. These contracts are made for a specific period of time (e.g., 1 week or 1 month) and must be renewed and renegotiated at the completion of the time period. Behavioral contracts have some success in a small group of adolescent users; however, their underlying success is related to the willingness of the teenager to use the device. Without it, the contract falls apart very rapidly.

Enlisting the aid of the school psychologist or guidance counselor may be necessary to understand the fundamental reasons behind the adolescent's decision to give up wearing the implant full time or on a limited basis. If the speech pathologist and teacher can work in conjunction with the psychologist, information can be shared to help enlighten all the professionals treating the teenager. Unfortunately, there are some cases in which the adolescent eventually refuses to wear the device at any time. After exhausting all alternatives, the professionals and the parents must accept this decision. Interestingly, there have been cases in which the adolescent has returned to partial use after years of nonuse, once he has completed high school and entered the workplace.

The Nonuser

Communication between the cochlear implant recipient and the implant facility, even for a "nonuser," is important because there may be a time when the individual decides to use his implant once again. However, if the processor has not been adjusted in several years, the settings for the implant are likely inappropriate and may create a negative response. Therefore, it behooves implant facilities to maintain an ongoing dialogue with the limited or nonuser. Too often, these recipient's names are removed from the mailing lists of the implant facilities because the majority of information being sent to other users is inappropriate. Regardless, nonusers should be contacted on a regular basis concerning their implant. Most important, reminders about the need for retuning the processor should be sent if nonusers decide to wear the device again.

Networking

The need to be in communication with other individuals with cochlear implants is greatest in the adolescent population. Contact with other teenagers who have been long-term users or short-term users is a means of providing this group with support from those with whom they share a common bond. The use of the TTY and the relay system has opened the world to deaf teenagers. Computer technology with the use of the FAX modem and Internet services now allow hearing-impaired individuals the ability to communicate at the stroke of a key. Recently, the A. G. Bell Association and Oticon Inc. established a teenage bulletin board utilizing electronic mail (E-mail), which will enable this group to interact more easily. All of this is a concerted effort to reach out to a population of deaf children who are struggling to find themselves.

Parents of teenagers often welcome any help they are offered. The years that are traditionally filled with confusion and lack of communication do not have to pass with tension and anxiety. Implanted teenagers who have approached the process with realistic expectations and have the support of their families and the proper professionals have maximized the benefits of wearing their devices. They remain a resource for other teenagers contemplating implantation as well as those who choose not to undergo the process.

■□ SUMMARY

The adolescent who has received a cochlear implant must be fully aware of the long-term commitment necessary in order to obtain maximal use of the device. Professionals who direct the therapy for this group of nonyoungsters (or nonadults) need to be cognizant of their interests, needs, and fears in order to drive the process to completion. In addition to the focused listening and speaking activities which need to take place, ongoing counseling is crucial to success. At times, this counseling may be outside the realm of the teacher or speech pathologist. In those instances, it is important for personnel who see the child on a regular basis to refer to the properly trained professional when the case demands specific attention. In the long term, adolescents who are treated with their individual needs in mind can be successful cochlear implant users, despite the fact that they may never attain open set speech recognition abilities.

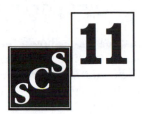

Performance of Children with Cochlear Implants

As with hearing aids, children who receive cochlear implants do not perform in a uniform fashion. This is not an unusual finding given the heterogeneous nature of the hearing-impaired population. Factors which contribute to the success of cochlear implantation include age of onset of deafness, duration of deafness, and age at implantation. There may be other contributing factors which are physiological in nature, such as neural supply or central processing abilities (Boothroyd, 1993). Additionally, research has demonstrated that access to good auditory training/learning also results in improved performance (Geers & Moog, 1991). It is important for the teacher in the classroom to understand the range of performance implanted children will exhibit, how that performance may change over time, and how to utilize to their advantage the support services which are available.

■□ AUDITORY PERCEPTION
WITH COCHLEAR IMPLANTS

Studies have shown that all children who receive a cochlear implant and wear it on a full-time basis demonstrate some improvement in their auditory perceptual abilities (Osberger et al., 1991b; Staller et al.,1991; Tyler, 1993). The assessment of these abilities is achieved across the hierarchy of perception which spans detection, discrimination, identification, and comprehension (see Chapter 7).

Linguistically appropriate materials for children of differing age groups have been used for purposes of measuring change in performance over time. As a practicality, this change in performance is obtained through the use of test materials which have been developed using conventional hearing aids and tactile aids as well as cochlear implants. These test materials have been standardized on a population of hearing-impaired children. These procedures fall into two basic categories known as closed set and open set measures of speech perception.

Closed Set Measures of Speech Perception

Closed set measures of speech perception include those test materials in which the choices of the stimuli being presented are provided to the child. The number of choices available to the child can be as few as two or many more. Depending on which perceptual task is being tapped, the stimuli might vary according to word patterns (cat vs. ice cream cone) or phonemes (pat vs. bat). Regardless of which level of perceptual performance is under scrutiny, children are presented with the printed words, pictures which depict the words, or the actual objects themselves. The task requires the child to select one of the items after each presentation; thus, no verbal response is required. Ambiguous responses are not possible. The child must always choose one of the items available to him. Since there is always the possibility the child may randomly select the correct response, closed set tests require that a chance score be calculated. This chance score will depend on the number of choices available for each presentation. It is important for teachers/therapists reviewing information concerning a particular child's performance to understand the relationship between the chance score and the actual score. For example, in a closed set test with only two choices, a chance score of 50% would be computed. If a child scored 60% on a test such as this, the majority of his score should be viewed as being a function of chance. If, however, the same child scored similarly on a closed set test in which the chance score was 20%, his score could be viewed as representing relatively good performance on the skill which the test was evaluating.

Closed set tests are used across the entire age range of child implant users. For very young children, this is most often the only method of obtaining some response measures. It is important for teachers and therapists who review reports from cochlear implant facilities that the types of tests administered be clearly distinguished. Common closed set tests for this population include the Monosyllable, Trochee, Spondee Test (MTS) (Erber & Alencewicz, 1976), the Early Speech Perception Battery (ESP) (Moog & Geers, 1990), and the Northwestern University Children's Perception of Speech Test (Nu-Chips) (Elliot & Katz, 1980). A complete description of these and other closed set tests can be found in Appendix H.

Open Set Measures of Speech Perception

Open set measures of speech perception are more difficult than closed set measures because the possible responses are not provided to the child. These are the more standard types of audiological procedures utilized for everyday evaluation of hearing impairment. Traditionally, these procedures use single syllable word or sentence stimuli which the child must repeat after each presentation. For example, children with measurable hearing are often given word lists known as the Phonetically Balanced Kindergarten Test (PBKs) (Haskins, 1949). These are phonetically balanced single syllable words representative of a normal hearing child's vocabulary at the kindergarten level. The audiologist asks the child to "Say the word _____." The child's score represents the number of words correctly repeated from a list of 50. The linguistic constraints of the child may contribute to his ability to perform this type of task. For example, children with restricted vocabulary may appear to perform poorer than usual because they have a limited number of words in their lexicon. Additionally, a child must have intelligible speech so that the individual evaluating performance is certain of the correct response.

Substantial open set speech recognition obtained using auditory input alone is the standard for which evaluators of all types of auditory prostheses strive. Effectively, if a child is able to obtain a significant amount of open set speech recognition, he is processing information in an auditory-only modality. This is no small feat for a profoundly deaf child. A listing of open set tests of speech perception can be found in Appendix I.

◨ SPEECHREADING ASSESSMENT

Although the ultimate goal of cochlear implantation is to provide enough auditory input to the child to decrease his dependence on speechreading, this is not always possible. Some assessment of the child's speechreading ability should be performed pre- and postoperatively in order to measure changes in this skill area. Many of the closed set tests are often performed initially in a visual-plus-auditory mode. This provides the child with an opportunity to review the materials on the test, and it affords the evaluator an estimate of the child's speechreading skill. Depending on the child's linguistic level, single word, sentence material, or connected sentences can be used. For the very young child with limited language, the "body parts" test is often administered. This requires the child to point to the body part which is named by the evaluator. For the child with more sophisticated linguistic skills, traditional methods of speechtracking using simple stories can be used. Speechtracking (DeFillipo & Scott, 1978) requires the child to repeat, verbatim, sentences in a story which are being read aloud. The ability to perform this task is dependent on the child's knowledge of the language and his own speech production intelligibility.

The speechreading component of the evaluation supplies information about the child's ability to understand speech when visual cues are made available. For children with some degree of linguistic competence, it demonstrates the child's communicative ability in a face-to-face situation. Speechreading teaches the child to utilize the auditory signal to differentiate sounds which look alike on the face (Tye-Murray, 1992). Even if a comprehensive evaluation of speechreading is not possible because of language constraints, the presentation of stimuli with visual cues assesses the child's understanding of the functional components of the speech act. Practically, it answers the question as to whether the child has a realization that movement of the speaker's mouth has certain ramifications with regard to communication.

◨ SPEECH PERCEPTION CHANGES

The large mass of cochlear implant data (Osberger et al., 1991b; Staller et al., 1991; Tyler et al., 1986) have been obtained using a single subject, repeated measures design. This requires that a baseline measure be obtained prior to implantation and that each child act as his own control. Because all children in the data pool did not receive all the same tests, the test procedures were classified into groups of categories that were representative of certain speech perceptual abilities. For example, the Monosyllable Trochee Spondee Test (MTS) taps the same types of auditory perceptual abilities as the Early Speech Perception Test (ESP). The major difference between these two procedures is related to the specific words used for each test. Younger children may not be capable of performing the MTS test due to limitations in their vocabulary. Both tests, however, measure the child's ability to discriminate words based on timing and intensity cues and understand words in a closed set format. Thus, the interpretation of their scores can be compared.

To assist in grouping the data more easily to measure changes over time, categories of speech perception, which were already in use when assessing deaf children (Geers & Moog, 1987), were expanded on. These speech perception categories were originally developed as factors contributing to the ability to predict the development of spoken language. Initially, four categories existed. The field of cochlear implants has contributed to the identification of a fifth (and sometimes sixth) category.

Category 1 (No Pattern Perception) represents those children who are unable to make judgments about the various word or sentence patterns presented in an auditory-only mode. These children are unable to differentiate between a single syllable word (or nonsense syllable) and a multisyllable word (or nonsense syllable). For example, the child is not capable of distinguishing the difference between the word cat versus ice cream cone or ba versus ba-ba-ba based solely on their differences in durational cues.

For the teacher in the classroom, this would mean that the child would be unable to make simple discriminations based on the patterns of sounds. Because the child is unable to make these discriminations, more often than not, this same child will probably show inconsistent or limited alerting responses to sound. Most children who receive cochlear implants are classified as Category 1 at the preoperative stage. Postoperatively, with rare exception, children quickly move from this category to the next.

Category II (Pattern Perception) includes those children who are able to discriminate sound based on an ability to differentiate patterns. These timing and/or intensity cues are used to make the discrimination that one sound is different from the other. Timing or durational cues refer to the temporal characteristics of the sound. For example a sound may occur for a brief period of time (microwave oven beeping) or may occur over a longer period (running water). These timing cues can be classified into signals which are long versus short, continuous versus interrupted or single versus multisyllable.

Intensity cues include those signals which vary according to the relative loudness of one signal to the next, that is, a soft sound (or syllable) versus a loud sound (or syllable). The combination of these cues aids in the discriminability of spoken words. Teachers with students who are able to discriminate sounds based on the perception of speech patterns should have an understanding of how this ability will impact on their classroom performance. These children should be able to discriminate a variety of environmental sounds as well as detect their names. These responses may not be spontaneous and may only occur when there is a great deal of structure. For children with more sophisticated language levels, the addition of information obtained from detecting speech patterns will enhance the ability to speechread. Thus, pattern recognition will facilitate communication between the teacher and the student when the child has access to visual cues and is being spoken to on a linguistic level for which he has some competence.

Category III (Some Word Recognition) is a higher level of functioning which requires the child to identify and recognize words when presented in an auditory-only modality. Children who reach this level of performance demonstrate an ability which is often the foundation for the development of open set speech recognition. This ability, however, is neither consistent nor generalizable across speaker-listener situations. Teachers with children in their classroom who are classified as Category III performers find oral communication easier than with children in Categories I and II. The teacher may notice that the child's ability to speechread occurs with greater facility than children in the other two prior categories. However, visual cues are still necessary for communication and some repetition of the spoken word may be required at times.

Category IV (Consistent Word Recognition) includes that group of children who are able to consistently understand *known* speech stimuli without visual cues. These children are able to perform better in situations in which there is some knowledge of the topic or words in use. Although these children continue to speechread, conversation is much more free flowing, and there are fewer repetitions necessary for understanding. For example, the teacher may discover that children in this category are able to understand previously reviewed spelling words without having to look up from their paper. Again, speechreading is necessary for maximal communication but the overall communication exchange is easier.

Category V (Open Set Word Recognition) comprises those children who are capable of understanding speech without the aid of speechreading. These are children who do not need to see the speaker's face in order to understand the content of the message. Teachers of children with Category V speech perception ability find that visual cues are not necessarily required for understanding. It is important, however, to realize that because the teacher may be introducing new ideas and concepts, speechreading is still necessary to ensure comprehension. Even though these children display a significant amount of open set speech recognition ability, the teacher should not be misled into thinking that the child hears normally. Strategies which foster good communication should continue to be implemented; that is, new information should be presented under the best communication situations.

Some centers have instituted a Category VI which is meant to include those children whose open set speech recognition is more consistent than those in Category V. Regardless, children in either Categories V or VI demonstrate an ability to understand speech without the aid of visual cues. A summary of these speech perception categories can be found in Table 11–1.

■□ ANALYSIS OF RESULTS

The largest body of data concerning the performance of children using cochlear implants has been collected by Cochlear Corporation, the manufacturer of the Nucleus device. This data collection was per-

TABLE 11–1
Speech Perception Categories

Category 1	No Pattern Perception
Category 2	Pattern Perception
Category 3	Some Word Identification
Category 4	Consistent Word Identification
Category 5	Open Set Word Recognition

Source: From Geers, A. E., & Moog, J. S. (1987). Predicting spoken language acquisition in profoundly deaf children. *Journal of Speech and Hearing Disorders 52*, pp. 84–94.

formed as part of the premarket approval process required by the Food and Drug Administration. As of June 1995, the Nucleus device is the only device to have received premarket approval for use in the pediatric population. Worldwide there have been over 4,000 implants performed in children. Approximately 1,500 of these have taken place in the United States (Cochlear Corporation, personal communication, January, 1995). The data collected to obtain FDA approval were gathered on 142 children who were followed for a minimum of 2 years. Over time, the accrual of data has continued for this original group of subjects as well as newly implanted children. Since premarket approval of the device, the number of cochlear implant surgeries has increased substantially. Staller and colleagues (1991), Osberger and colleagues (1991b), and Tyler (1993) have published the results of studies that have measured changes in performance in children with cochlear implants. For purposes of this chapter, these data will be interpreted to reflect the *functional* performance changes in children with implants and how these changes might affect the teaching style in the classroom.

Auditory Perceptual Changes in the Very Young Implanted Child

Children who are congenitally deaf or early deafened and are implanted within 2 to 3 years of age have exhibited substantial improvement with continued implant use. Data indicate that if these children are placed in programs that value audition and spoken language, they are more likely to develop open set speech recognition (Category V/VI) (Waltzman, Cohen, & Shapiro, 1994). The majority of these children begin with auditory abilities classified as either Category I or II. Although some children are in normal preschool environments with teachers who have had no exposure to hearing-impaired children, many are in self-contained classrooms (Nevins & Chute, 1994). Expectations of teachers with these children in their classrooms may vary widely. Experience with the child prior to the time of the implant will provide the teacher with a baseline of auditory functioning so that his improvements in auditory abilities are appreciated. Teachers without prior experience with the child may expect him to be capable of more sophisticated responses at too early a stage. Generally, it takes approximately 12–18 months of implant use before the child will exhibit consistent discrimination of speech sounds (Category III/IV).

Often, these auditory behaviors are directly related to the child's linguistic proficiency and develop in conjunction with it (Waltzman et al., 1994). Some behaviors develop more rapidly, however, including the ability of the child to detect his name and to discriminate environmental sounds. These responses are likely to be demonstrated within the first 6 months of implant use, provided the child is wearing the device on a full time basis (Osberger et al., 1991b; Staller et al., 1991). Children who were considered Category I (No Pattern Perception) prior to implantation will generally move into Category II (Pattern Perception) at a rapid rate, as long as the task is presented within a structured listening environment. Teachers should ensure that the child is always within visual proximity to enhance communication. As the child continues with his implant use, he will progress through the various speech perception categories. Frequently, children who are implanted at this young age participate in both self-contained classes and normal nursery classes during the course of their school day (Nevins & Chute, 1994). The self-contained program directs the language and speech instruction, whereas the preschool program provides the opportunity for socialization with hearing agemates.

Clearly, if the child is implanted at age 2 or 3 and it requires at least 12–18 months of implant use before significant changes occur, it is rare that the early infant or preschool teacher will observe the final results of the implantation process. It is more than likely that these teachers may experience some negative responses from the child (e.g., reluctance to wear the processor) and observe only limited gains which occur during this time. Lack of feedback from the child should not discourage the teacher during this vital period, for she is laying the foundation for future development of auditory and speech skills. Throughout this habilitative phase, the teacher should encourage listening behaviors and provide the child with an auditory enriched environment. Enthusiasm and a positive attitude will help foster good relationships among the child, the teacher, and his parents.

Speech Production Changes

Speech production changes for the greater majority of implanted children progress at much slower rates (Tobey, Geers, & Brenner, 1994). Because the development of intelligible speech is so closely linked to hearing ability, children implanted at an early age have the potential to develop more natural sounding and understandable speech than children implanted in their later years (Osberger, Robbins, Todd, & Riley, 1994). Although, the benefits provided by the implant should contribute to the articulation of more precise speech, the child's production will not change as rapidly as his perception. Teachers and parents who stress the use of speech in the class and at home will find that implanted children will demonstrate improvement at a quicker rate than those in classrooms and homes which do not.

Children Implanted at Ages 3–5 Years

The majority of the children in this age range will achieve results similar to those of the early implanted child, in that most will ultimately obtain open set speech recognition (Category V/VI) (Brackett & Zara, 1994; Waltzman et al, 1994). For children who are perilinguistically deafened (i.e., deafened between the ages of 2–5) performance changes will vary. For those children with a significant amount of language prior to their loss of hearing, the advances will be more rapid than for those who had limited linguistic abilities at the onset of deafness. For example, a child born with normal hearing and normal language development who lost his hearing following meningitis at age 4 will progress quickly when implanted at age 5. In contrast, a child who is deafened at age 2 with very limited language prior to the loss of hearing and implanted at age 5 will exhibit a slower rate of improvement (Parisier & Chute, 1994). The major difference between these two children is related to the duration of deafness each sustained. Generally, as the duration of deafness increases, the achieved performance level of the child may be less (Osberger et al., 1994). In the examples listed above, the child with the shorter duration of deafness will progress more quickly and achieve higher levels than the second child. However, because both children are relatively young and within the language-learning years at the time of implantation, the overall results with both children are often good (Gantz, Tyler, Woodworth, Tye-Murray, & Fryauf-Bertschy, 1994).

The classroom teacher of a 5-year-old congenitally deaf child will usually observe a marked change in behavior regarding sound detection within the first 6 months of implant use. However, word recognition behavior (Category III) may not be exhibited for at least another 6–12 months of implant use for a child with this profile (Staller, Beiter, & Brimacombe, 1994).

Speech production changes in children who are pre/perilinguistically deafened with long durations of deafness (e.g., children deafened at 13 months and implanted at age 5) will follow a much slower course than those children who had developed speech skills prior to losing their hearing (Osberger et al., 1994). The teacher may notice that although the child may be performing relatively well in the auditory perceptual domain, his speech production has not changed significantly during that same period. This is quite typical of this group and should not be viewed as indicative of low performance. In time, the speech production will progress, as long as the child is being trained and challenged to use this modality.

For the child with a short duration of deafness, development of consistent word recognition skills (Category IV) may appear within the first year of receiving the implant. In many cases, children who have had good language development prior to losing their hearing exhibit open set speech recognition ability after approximately 12 to 18 months of implant use (Gantz et al., 1994). Teachers of children with this type of hearing history should observe marked changes in their ability to perceive speech and attend in class.

The speech production changes observed for this group will often be dependent on the skill level of the child prior to his loss of hearing. Interestingly, however, even this group of children will often display a dramatic deterioration of their productive abilities soon after the hearing loss. This occurs as a result of the lack of auditory feedback during a time when the child is still developing his speech skills. It is not unusual to find children who have lost most of their speech after the onset of deafness, despite the fact that they were speaking appropriately prior to the loss (Economou, Tartter, Chute, & Hellman, 1992).

Children Implanted at Ages 5–8 Years

Children in this age group who are postlinguistically deafened with short durations of deafness perform extremely well and at a rapid rate. These children often attain open set speech recognition skills within the first 9 to 18 months of implant use (Staller et al., 1994). If there has been any deterioration in speech production skills prior to implantation, generally these skills rebound quickly. The teachers of a child with this hearing history may notice marked changes immediately following implantation, along with steady progress over time. Some of these children may have been removed from the mainstream prior to implantation. Once their auditory and speech skills have returned, often they are able to make the transition to the regular classroom

(Nevins & Chute, 1994). Teachers, however, should realize that despite the child's new auditory capabilities, it is always best to provide him with as much visual input as necessary to facilitate learning.

Children in this age group who are pre/perilinguistically deafened will demonstrate achievement at a much slower rate (Gantz et al., 1994). The teacher should remember, once again, that as the duration of deafness increases, the level of performance reached with the implant may be limited and occurs at a reduced rate of growth. These children will often attain Category III (Some Word Recognition) and IV (Consistent Word Recognition) capabilities after 1½–3 years of implant experience. Depending on the age of onset of the deafness relative to the age at the time of implantation (i.e., duration of deafness), fewer numbers of these children will obtain open set speech recognition abilities.

Speech production changes in older implanted children with long durations of deafness will lag comparatively to children with short durations of deafness. Tobey (1993) reported that 13% of young children and 50% of older children showed clinical improvement for segmental imitation tasks. However, overall speech intelligibility of children with longer durations of deafness may be a function of the abilities attained prior to implantation, their access to adequate training, and the duration of implant use (Gantz et al., 1994). Children in this group may require years of implant use before the actual merits of the device contribute to their speech. For this group and those in older groups, the data that are available at this time may not reflect the final performance. There may be the potential for children in this age group to demonstrate greater benefit after many years of using the implant.

Children Implanted after the Age of 8 Years

Because it is evident that the child who is postlinguistically deafened will generally perform at a superior rate and level, it is not necessary to continue to describe this group. Children implanted above the age of 8 who are pre/perilinguistically or congenitally deaf are not likely to attain open set speech recognition. There are always exceptions to this (Sarant, Cowan, Blamey, Galvin, & Clark, 1994); however, the majority of the early deafened and late implanted children will progress to Category III and IV only after years of experience. This becomes especially important when considering the implantation of congenitally deaf or early deafened teenagers. The major impact of the cochlear implant on this age group is in speechreading improvement and environmental sound discrimination (Chute, 1993). Changes in these areas can have a positive effect on the child's ability to function in the classroom, making communication and the transmission of information easier for both the teacher and the student. Expectations of teachers of children in this age group should be realistic and supportive. These children should not be expected to function without the aid of visual cues, nor should major gains in speech production be anticipated. However, as noted above, this group may require much longer periods of implant use before their performance reaches asymptote. Recent data from facilities that have implanted and followed these children for more than 5 years indicate that these children are still making progress albeit slowly (Gantz et al., 1994; Osberger et al., 1994).

■ SPECIAL POPULATIONS

There are special groups of children who receive cochlear implants who may not follow the general performance trends that have been described. These groups include children who have partial insertions of their cochlear implants, children who may have been born with severe hearing losses and later developed profound hearing losses, children with borderline responses with hearing aids prior to implantation, and children with multiple handicaps. It is important for the teacher to have a knowledge of whether the child in class is a member of one of these groups, because these children tend to follow a different pattern of performance over time.

Partial Insertions

Children who have a partial insertion of their cochlear implant are generally children who have had meningitis or present with a malformed cochlea (often known as a Mondini deformity). Children who have had meningitis often experience an abnormal amount of bone growth (ossification) on the cochlea. Ossified cochleas result in a hardening of the bone and the membranes in the cochlea, which prevents the surgeon from passing the electrode completely (Gantz, McCabe, & Tyler, 1988). In children with Mondini deformities, the cochlea has not fully developed into its complete 2½ turns and, therefore, cannot house the entire electrode array. A knowledge of how children in each of these groups respond with a cochlear implant will be helpful to the classroom teacher and therapists working with them.

Ossified Cochleas

In cases of partial insertions due to ossification of the cochlea, the surgeon is usually able to implant 10 electrodes. These electrodes are not necessarily inserted into the membranes of the cochlea but rather are laid in a trough drilled out at the time of the surgery. This differs substantially from traditional cochlear implant surgery. Physically, the membranes of the normal cochlea usually contain fluid which has a certain chemical composition. This chemical composition contributes to the inductance of the electrical activity that is generated when an electrode is activated. Without this chemical solution surrounding the electrode it often will necessitate the use of more current to generate a response (Parisier & Chute, 1993). Also, the thickness of the bone which has grown in the cochlea will restrict the amount of current needed to excite the nerve endings. Finally, because the number of electrodes is restricted, it is not possible to deliver the electrical information in the same manner as when there is a full insertion with 22 electrodes implanted. Thus, children with partial insertions due to ossified cochleas have a limited number of electrodes available for stimulation and generally (but not in all cases) require large amounts of current to produce a reaction.

When the number of electrodes is restricted, the frequency bands assigned to each of the electrodes is larger so that the ability to make finer discriminations may be jeopardized. Studies regarding children with partial insertions have reported a variety of results (Kemink, Zimmerman-Phillips, Kileny, Firszt, & Novak, 1992; Parisier & Chute, 1993). Parisier and Chute (1993) reported on five children with partial insertions who demonstrated progress at much slower rates and often did not attain speech perception abilities commensurate with their age and duration of deafness. Often, these children will exhibit inconsistent responses to sound for the first 12–18 months. In many cases, the children do not progress past Category II (Pattern Perception) performance. Conversely, Kemink et al. (1992) and Zimmerman-Phillips, Firszt, and Kileny (1990) found performance similar to those with full insertions; however, in some cases these responses were observed after years of implant use. Research regarding speech production changes for this subgroup has not been systematically performed nor compared to the general population of implant users.

Often, teachers of children who have partial insertions due to cochlear ossification will note a great deal of inconsistency and lack of response from the child for as long as a year after implantation (Geier, Gilden, Luetje, & Maddox, 1993). It is best to encourage the child by setting up structured listening situations which are time locked and foster success. Constant communication with the implant center will assist the teacher in coping with the limited responses. Although open set speech recognition may not be initially forthcoming, children with partial insertions obtain substantial visual enhancement of the speech signal which eases the communication exchange (Kirk, Sehgal, & Miyamoto, in press).

Mondini Deformities

Electrical responses of children with Mondini deformities are vastly different from children with ossified cochleas despite the fact that in many cases, there is only a partial insertion of the array. Although the medical literature classifies these types of deformities more specifically depending on how much of the cochlea is absent, the nonmedical literature groups them together under one general term. The reader should be made aware that some children with this deformity may have only one turn to their cochlea, whereas others may not have a cochlea at all. Children with malformed cochleas often exhibit threshold and comfort levels that fluctuate frequently, especially during the early months post tune-up. These fluctuations in T and C levels create inconsistent responses to sound, because there are times the device is not delivering enough current (and therefore sound is not audible) and other times when it is delivering too much current (and sound is too loud). Oftentimes, these children must return to the implant center for more frequent retunes to accommodate these changes. Responses of children with Mondini deformities are directly related to the degree of the deformity (i.e., how much of the cochlea is actually present). In some children with almost two full turns to the cochlea, the results can be comparable to other children with similar ages and durations of deafness. Even as the degree of the malformation increases, children are capable of utilizing the signal from the implant to obtain an enhancement in speechreading ability (Novak, Firszt, Brown, & Reeder, 1990; Firszt, Reeder, & Novak, in press).

For teachers of children who have partial insertions due to Mondini deformities, there must be a heightened awareness if responses suddenly cease or if there are complaints of the device being too loud. This, generally, is indicative of the child's need for a remapping of the speech processor. Expectations for performance must be considered with a number of interacting variables. Performance (in the areas of speech perception and speech production) for this group may be a function of the child's age at the time of implantation and the duration of deafness (as with all groups of implant users) and the number of electrodes inserted (as it is related to the extent of the malformation).

Children with Progressive Hearing Losses

There is a group of children which includes individuals who have been hearing impaired from birth but not profoundly hearing impaired since that time. Generally, these are children who present with moderately severe sensorineural hearing losses which respond well to traditional amplification. These children are amplified early, remediated, and often in mainstream school environments. Occasionally, and for unknown reasons, a small percentage of these children will suddenly experience a large decrement in their hearing abilities, thereby placing them into the profoundly deaf category. The issues facing these children, parents, and their teachers are quite different from anything discussed thus far.

Sometimes, this decrease in hearing sensitivity occurs during the preteen or teenage years. These years, in and of themselves, present with difficulties even for normal hearing children. The progression to a profound loss may take place suddenly or may occur over time, with fluctuations in hearing level. Regardless of how the progression to profound deafness has occurred, the child is often in a confused and anxious state auditorally, socially, and academically. The use of the acoustical amplification which had been successful for them is now found to be inadequate. The notion of a cochlear implant for these children may be viewed as a method of returning them to their prior state. However, acoustical amplification is substantially different from electrical stimulation and often their expectations are unrealized.

Initially, there is frequent disappointment for the child, because the sounds from the cochlear implant are markedly different from sounds they obtained with their hearing aids. Additionally, the expectations for immediate recovery to their previous level of performance are often unrealistic despite aggressive counseling by the implant team. Teachers may also anticipate, erroneously, that the child will return to the level of functioning that he had prior to his loss, at a rate which is faster than possible. Counseling and communication, coupled with aggressive auditory training, is crucial to the success of children with progressive hearing loss.

Experience with these children at Manhattan Eye, Ear & Throat Hospital in New York suggests that the return of function for this group usually occurs within 6 months to 1 year postimplantation if implanted soon after the profound loss. The pattern and progress usually follows that of the postlinguistically deafened child; however, the final level achieved may vary. Most of the children will attain Category IV speech perception ability by the end of the first year of implant use. Development of Category V/VI ability will be child dependent and related to the preprofound level of achievement. More in-depth study of children in this group is needed to determine the implant's effects on both speech perception and production.

Teachers should recognize that children with progressive loss will not return to their prior functioning level immediately postimplantation. Listening activities require a relearning of sound through the new prosthesis. Therapists should not presume skill levels in areas in which the child was previously capable. Auditory lessons may necessitate a return to lower levels to ensure ability as well as foster success. Support for these children, especially in the early days post tune-up is critical. Data from a small group of children (N = 5) at Manhattan Eye, Ear & Throat Hospital demonstrate that most children in this group will return to their previous functioning level and, in many cases, eventually surpass it. Both, however, will take time.

Children with Borderline Responses with Hearing Aids

As children with cochlear implants demonstrate better responses, parents of children who have some residual hearing are questioning the use of this device for their own children. Many professionals, as well as parents, note that children with relatively good responses with hearing aids in the low and mid frequencies are still unable to discriminate or produce high frequency sounds with good consistency (Brackett & Zara, 1994). Oftentimes, these children are able to perform well in structured evaluations; however, they are unable to perform in a similar fashion in more natural settings or when the speaker is beyond a close range (Zimmerman-Phillips et al., 1994).

Preoperatively, this group of children is capable of demonstrating performance which is classified as Category II, III, and in some cases IV when tested under controlled conditions (Skinner, 1994). Practically, however, the children are often unable to perform to this level with great consistency on a daily basis. Although their speech production skills may also have a high degree of intelligibility, there remain large portions of unintelligible sequences, especially when the context is unknown (Brackett & Zara, 1994). Decisions regarding implantation of children with this type of profile must be carefully weighed. The role of the educational consultant is important to the assessment of such children. Observations over time occurring in naturalistic settings, such as the classroom or at home, must be made to determine the candidacy of these children. Assessing children at a variety of sound pressure levels may also be helpful in determining candidacy (Skinner, 1994; Zimmerman-Phillips et al., 1994). Counseling the parents regarding the final outcome is also vital.

Overall, the results of studies on speech perception and speech production abilities in children with residual hearing who use a cochlear implant suggest performance which is superior to children who use amplification for this level of hearing. The initial studies reported by Osberger et al. (1991b) assessed cochlear implant performance comparing it to a range of hearing aid users. Those with residual hearing who had cochlear implants outperformed those with residual hearing who used traditional amplification.

The small body of literature pertaining to speech production changes following implantation of children with residual hearing has been slower to materialize. Nonetheless, there is every indication that children in this group who receive implants demonstrate improvement in speech production faster than the traditional implant user and equivalent to the good users of hearing aids (Brackett & Zara, 1994; Tobey et al., 1994).

Children with Multiple Handicaps

Although children with multiple handicaps represent a small subset of the cochlear implant population, they do exist. Children with Usher Syndrome or Retinitis Pigmentosa are both profoundly deaf and visually impaired. Often the profound deafness is the initial problem with the deterioration of vision occurring later. In some children, the visual problems may begin as early as 6 years of age, whereas in others the visual problems do not develop until they are young adults. The performance of children with Usher syndrome follow the same patterns as those in the general pediatric cochlear implant population; that is, children who are implanted early with shorter durations of deafness tend to perform better (Chute & Nevins, 1995). However, because a child with a diagnosis of Usher Syndrome will eventually also lose vision, it is important that professionals evaluating children for implantation consider this factor during the rehabilitation period.

Many of the effects of Usher Syndrome on the visual system are, at first, extremely subtle. Night blindness and tunnel vision may occur initially. This must be kept in mind when structuring support services for the child in the classroom and developing a program for auditory training. Sign language interpreters who are removed from the child's visual field are useless. Auditory activities that do not address environmental awareness will be less effective. The importance of informing teachers of the child's visual needs cannot be overlooked because many teachers of the deaf have little, if any, information about this subpopulation. Finally, the presence of Usher Syndrome in the profoundly deaf population should act as a reminder to clinicians and teachers to ensure proper evaluation of the visual system in conjunction with the auditory system.

The last group, although extremely limited in size, includes those children who exhibit cognitive deficits or autistic behaviors (Bellman, 1994; Lesinski et al., 1994). As a whole, these children achieve at the lower end of the performance spectrum with most obtaining only sound detection and a smaller number obtaining pattern perception. The poorest and most inconsistent group of performers are the children who have been diagnosed with autism. At this time, autistic children do not perform well enough to warrant implantation (Lesinski et al., 1994). In children who exhibit various levels of retardation, parents and professional report better behavior management overall and environmental awareness that address issues of safety (Bellman, 1994). Implantation of children in these special categories requires a more extensive team with members who have qualifications in areas of cognition, behavior management, and psychology.

■□ SUMMARY

Cochlear implantation in the pediatric population has produced results across a wide variety of children, which indicate successful use by the profoundly deaf. All children who wear their implants obtain some degree of benefit. The magnitude of change in both speech perception and speech production may vary according to physiological and environmental factors. Physiological factors address issues regarding the integrity of the cochlea, neural responsiveness, and the presence of other physical or cognitive involvement. Environ-mental factors include access to good auditory training and both parental and school support.

Teachers of implanted children need to be aware of all of the variables which interact with overall performance. They must be realistic with regard to the course of progress for an individual child in light of the larger performance characteristics of the pediatric population and its particular subgroups. Patience and support are key to providing the child with the opportunity to maximize benefit from the device.

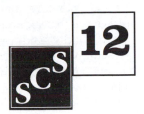

Mainstreaming and Children with Cochlear Implants

Society's responsibility is to educate its children. There are certain ideal conditions of the school environment and characteristics of the teacher/learner dyad which contribute to the successful fulfillment of this responsibility. First, the *environment* in which this education occurs should accommodate the individuality of the child, foster the development of a positive self-image, and provide the best academic curriculum. *Teachers* in ideal educational environments should appreciate the diversity of the children they teach, maintain a solid knowledge base regarding the numerous aspects of curriculum content, and reflect on their teaching practice in order to tailor it to the needs of the children in their classroom. *Children* should be enthusiastic learners who come to school with certain prerequisite skills and display a social maturity commensurate with age and school placement.

These conditions and attributes are applicable whether the academic environment is a regular school or a school for the deaf, whether teachers are certified in regular education or deaf education, and whether the children are hearing or not. Finding the best match between the child and the school placement is the primary objective of both the system and the family. Therefore, parents of children with special needs must be aggressive in seeking proper placement and management.

A child's needs and abilities should dictate the most appropriate educational environment in which learning can be maximized. Determining placement must be accomplished using established criteria to prevent a school system from making decisions based solely on economics and convenience. Additionally, safeguards within the system should preclude parents from making placement demands based solely on emotions and unrealistic expectations. Movement between and among placements should be guaranteed as the child's needs and abilities change. When schools and parents are cooperative partners in the decision-making process, it is likely that the child's best interests and special requirements will be realized. Facilitating that partnership may necessitate the services of an outside professional. This advocate for the child ensures that the system, the child, and the parent have explored all placement possibilities before making a final decision.

◼ THE DEAF CHILD AND SCHOOL PLACEMENTS

The continuum of school placements available for deaf children today is a result of historical and political forces. Some parents choose a placement which reflects a philosophical orientation and provides a specific linguistic and cultural environment. Often, this choice is made at the start of the child's school career and remains unchanged for his entire educational experience. Some parents are not active participants in the process and therefore the placement choice is decided by the district on the basis of expediency. Still other parents make educational placement choices for their child with the expectation that the placement will change over time. Movement along the continuum from placements considered to be *more restrictive* to those labeled *least restrictive* is often the goal of parents who seek the development of oral language skills for their children. This often means placement in classrooms with hearing children in the mainstream.

The traditional use of the word *mainstream* begs the question of social mainstreaming or academic mainstreaming. Often deaf children were "mainstreamed" for nonacademic activities, that is, art, gym, and music. This process was known as social mainstreaming and met with limited success depending on individual circumstances. Academic mainstreaming was reserved only for those children whose achievement qualified them for placement in the regular classroom. The attainment of mainstream status was regarded as an accomplishment which, unfortunately, often resulted in the loss of crucial support services. The new term, *inclusion* attempts to combine aspects of both social and academic mainstreaming. No longer are particular achievement levels required in the practice of full inclusion. Rather, special education services are provided *in* the regular classroom regardless of the child's academic functioning. For purposes of the following discussion, the term *mainstreaming* will continue to be used to identify children who are placed in general education settings. This usage suggests that these children meet certain academic standards for placement but at the same time receive the necessary support services.

There appears to be general consensus that mainstream placement is most appropriate for the hard of hearing child (Paul & Quigley, 1984; Ross, Brackett, & Maxon, 1991). Although placement of the young profoundly deaf child in a mainstream classroom does not occur with great frequency, the availability of cochlear implant technology makes it a more reachable social and academic goal. Despite this fact, the concept of mainstreaming profoundly deaf students has both its supporters and detractors. Some view placement with hearing peers in a school setting as the ultimate educational objective for the profoundly deaf child (Manning, 1990). Others argue that the mainstream is not the least restrictive environment but is a more *communicatively* restricted environment than special class placement (Johnson et al., 1989). There are certain advantages ascribed to the mainstream setting, however, which make it a viable placement choice for deaf children.

■□ ADVANTAGES OF MAINSTREAM PLACEMENT

A number of performance characteristics of deaf children in the mainstream suggest an obvious advantage to mainstream placement, especially when considering academic achievement and speech production ability. Students placed in the mainstream attain higher levels on standardized tests of achievement than do their nonmainstreamed peers (Allen & Osborn, 1984; Pflaster, 1980). Speech intelligibility of children in mainstream settings is often superior to those in special education classes. Some have suggested that it is the lesser degree of hearing loss generally found in children in the mainstream which accounts for better speech intelligibility. It may also be that good speech intelligibility is part of the selection criteria for placement there. However, a third possibility is that students learn to articulate more clearly when they need to communicate with their hearing peers. Regardless, a decision of readiness for mainstream education is individual and must be made after considering a number of factors indicative of potential for success in the regular school setting.

■ REQUISITE SKILLS FOR GENERAL EDUCATION PLACEMENT

Appropriate placement in the mainstream can only be recommended if a "whole-child approach" to assessment has been utilized. For these purposes, the child must be evaluated using standardized tests which are normed on hearing children. Formal measures in the areas of language and reading must be obtained in order to predict how a child may perform when compared to his normal hearing peers. However, there are a number of informal indicators which can contribute to the identification of a child's readiness for the mainstream. These indicators include his academic standing in his present classroom, his ability to articulate his needs verbally, and his social interaction with other children. As for academic standing, the candidate for the mainstream should be at the top of his class, having been exposed to content curriculum commensurate with his age and grade level. This should enable a relatively easy transition from the self-contained to the mainstream classroom with hearing agemates. Oftentimes, summer tutoring which builds *curriculum-specific* background knowledge is essential to guarantee a child's ability to compete in the mainstream.

The candidate should have good speech intelligibility, demonstrating simple conversational competence. This conversational competence should be demonstrated using acquired oral skills so that child-child and teacher-child communication can take place directly. There are some children in mainstream environments as a result of academic needs and abilities. These children may use sign as their primary mode of communication and have limited oral skills. Often, they rely upon an interpreter to facilitate conversation in the classroom. They may become socially isolated because of their inability to communicate directly with other students and teachers. Finally, when a deaf child has a positive self-image, mainstream success from a social perspective is a greater possibility. Children with a positive self-image are able to define themselves by other individual attributes and not by their deafness. The child may be socially outgoing or popular with other children because of a special sports ability or talent. This may ease acceptance in the mainstream.

In addition to evaluating the child's prerequisite skills, there are certain requisite responsibilities that must be met by the child's receiving school. First and foremost, a commitment to providing the educational services required by the child must be made. In many circumstances, this dictates the presence of qualified personnel to provide direct support to both the student and staff. Often, modifications in teaching style must be made to accommodate the deaf child in the classroom. Unless teachers are willing to change, they should not be given the responsibility for mainstream children. Supplementary services, including those of an oral or sign language interpreter, a teacher/tutor or tutor/notetaker, and a speech-language pathologist must be accessible, if necessary.

Adaptations of the physical setting may also be requested to create the best acoustic environment for the deaf child (Berg, 1987). Classroom noise has a deleterious effect on the child's ability to listen and process new and familiar information. Minor alterations to existing classrooms may make them more suitable for instruction of the deaf child. These may include carpeting, window treatments, and lighting adjustments. The receiving school should indicate its willingness to make these changes as well.

Some classroom teachers may identify themselves as amenable to working with a deaf child in their classroom. Often, these teachers are experienced veterans who are interested in the challenge of educating a child with special needs. Others may be identified by school administration based on their teaching record and style. Regardless, the teacher who is well-suited for a deaf child is one who is willing to make adjustments in teaching style to accommodate the child's needs. These are individuals who are committed to teaching as a profession and can adapt mandated curriculum to suit the child. Teachers such as these provide the best match for deaf children who meet the individual requirements for placement in the mainstream.

The traditional route to the regular classroom suggests that a child is able to develop entry level skills for mainstream placement after a "required" period of time in self-contained classes. Given the technology of the cochlear implant, however, the threshold of skills may need to be adjusted, especially when considering the very young implant recipient. It might be appropriate to recommend mainstream nursery placement with both direct and indirect support services for a 2½ year old. These support services should be provided by a teacher of the deaf to the child and to the regular nursery school staff. The services for the child should include individual speech, language, and auditory "lessons." These individual sessions should be provided on a daily basis for 30-minute periods. The content of these lessons are driven by the regular preschool curriculum and provide the student with an opportunity to preview or review the specific vocabulary and language of these lessons (see Chapter 8). Direction to the preschool staff should include suggestions for incorporating the concept of auditory learning into the daily activities of the classroom.

There is also evidence to suggest that deaf children receiving implants at an early age tend to enter the mainstream or less restrictive educational settings sooner than has been traditionally reported (Chute & Nevins, 1994). Therefore, there is a greater possibility that many more deaf children will find their way into the regular classroom during the preschool and early elementary years. Teachers who traditionally had little exposure to this population may suddenly find themselves at a loss for how to manage their classes containing children with hearing impairment. A movement toward a policy of full inclusion of all children, regardless of their individual needs, may also result in the early, but sometimes inappropriate, placement of deaf children in the mainstream.

The cochlear implant does not eradicate the effects of profound hearing loss, it only mitigates them. Children still present with special needs, chief among them the understanding of idiomatic expressions, sophisticated vocabulary, and advanced grammatical structures of English. In some cases, in an attempt to garner support for mainstream placement, professionals may present a "rose-colored" picture of a child's abilities with a cochlear implant. Although it is true that many of these children have enhanced auditory skills, it should be understood that they remain hearing impaired and require instructional modifications to accommodate their language needs. Often, the alternative to mainstream placement for children successfully using cochlear implants is the self-contained classroom in which the content and pace of the academic curriculum may not be sufficiently challenging. For this reason, parents often seek mainstream placement for their child.

It is important to recognize that, once placed in the mainstream, children require constant monitoring to ensure success. A review of current practices suggests that once a receiving school is identified and a child is placed in the mainstream, he is seldom followed with the same intensity evidenced prior to the placement decision. It is a naive expectation to believe that comprehensive premainstreaming evaluation ensures subsequent social and academic success.

■ PERFORMANCE IN THE MAINSTREAM

The Clarke School for the Deaf, Northampton, Massachusetts, routinely contracts with local school districts to provide support to the mainstream placement of its deaf school graduates and other deaf students who contract for their services (Manning, 1990). This model suggests that monitoring mainstream performance in the classroom is essential to ensure success. At the Cochlear Implant Center at Manhattan Eye, Ear & Throat Hospital (CIC/MEETH), on-site observation and teacher interview are aspects of the follow-up assessment of the appropriateness of a child's mainstream placement both educationally and socially. To assist the educational consultants of the Implant Center in monitoring the mainstream success of children with cochlear implants, a mainstreaming checklist was developed by the staff at CIC/MEETH in collaboration with the Clarke School for the Deaf. This checklist, used as a guide to naturalistic, qualitative observation, also provides quantitative data and identifies behaviors believed to be indicators of mainstream success. These behaviors are evaluated on a scale which records minimal to maximal outcomes in both social and educational domains.

■ THE MAINSTREAM CHECKLIST

In completing the checklist, the observer records features of the classroom, including a physical diagram of the room and the target child's location in the room. The class size and the number of adults present is also recorded. The general style of the teacher/learner environment is noted—prompts in this category include teacher-directed lesson, group discussion, cooperative learning. In keeping with the collaborative consultation model recommended during candidacy, the educational consultant attempts to foster a cooperative relationship between the mainstream school and the implant facility. The presence of an implant team observer in the mainstream should not be viewed as a threat to the classroom teacher but rather as service to the local facility. The use of the checklist guides the educational consultant to observe both social and academic behavior in the mainstream setting (see Appendix J).

In addition to completing the mainstream checklist, the implant center's educational consultant interviews the classroom teacher and identifies support personnel and services received by children in the mainstream. Teachers complete a form which requires them to select a statement which best describes the student's classroom performance from a forced choice of the following five alternatives: (a) socially and academically successful in the classroom; (b) academically successful, but limited social interaction with other students; (c) socially accepted but having some academic problems; (d) having both social and academic challenges in the mainstream; and (e) unsuccessful in the mainstream—inappropriately placed. Finally, the teacher is asked to rate the child's performance compared to the other children in the class by placing him in one of four quartiles.

The completion of the mainstreaming checklist by the educational consultant assists in identifying the strengths and weaknesses of particular students in their educational settings. It also validates the placement decision for students experiencing success. It can be used to demonstrate lack of success to parents of students placed inappropriately in the mainstream. In addition, the checklist serves as a counseling tool for the consultant to identify areas in which the teacher can encourage movement along the continuum to more maximal performance.

◼️⃞ ADDITIONAL FACTORS CONTRIBUTING TO MAINSTREAM SUCCESS

Issues beyond those of the child's performance in the classroom may also contribute to mainstream success. When a child becomes an integral member of the school community, it is likely that social acceptance will follow. Every attempt should be made to encourage the deaf child to participate in classroom and afterschool activities. Teachers should not refrain from calling on the child in class for fear he may not hear or understand her. While there may be a need for repetitions to achieve communication, efforts to engage the child directly should be made. The teacher should not, however, make exaggerated exceptions to class requirements that single the deaf child out unnecessarily. Although the deaf child is not like every other child in the class, he will wish to be treated so. Special accommodations should not be so obvious to the child or to his classmates.

The teacher's role in fostering classroom friendships should not be overlooked. It is often helpful if the teacher can identify to the parents the child in the class who seems to be the most friendly toward the deaf child. Nurturing budding relationships can be accomplished by seating the children in close proximity to one another or placing them in cooperative groups for special projects. For older children, there have been instances in which hearing classmates become speechtracking partners to hearing-impaired implant users. In addition, when the implant user is also knowledgeable in sign language, sign clubs can be formed that meet during the recess portion of the lunch hour or after school.

Teachers may be asked to notify parents when special friendships seem to be forming so that the parents can follow up with afterschool or weekend play dates. Good home-school interaction can also assist the parent in ensuring that homework assignments and school announcements are communicated correctly. Teachers can set up a buddy system within the classroom so that every child has a classmate to whom he is responsible for helping with school assignments. In this way, the attention is not focused on the deaf child and his particular needs. Rather, it creates a good communication system applicable for the entire class. Parents may also take an active role in their child's educational experience through participation in PTA activities or volunteering in the library or lunch room. Regardless of the form that home-school contact takes, communication between parents and teachers is important, especially in circumstances in which the child has entered the mainstream at a young age.

■ SUMMARY

The impact of the cochlear implant on the field of deaf education is only beginning. Early trends seem to indicate the potential for earlier mainstream placement which has a concomitant impact on the field of regular education and society at large. True mainstreaming, in the sense of full participation in the mainstream of school and society, can only be accomplished if proper assessment and follow-up are components of the process. To experience mainstream success, the deaf child with a cochlear implant needs support. Who provides this support is unclear and often left unaddressed. Facilities committed to a comprehensive implant program must ensure that the educational issues are managed properly throughout the complex and ever changing process of implantation. Attending to the needs of the whole deaf child rather than simply the audiological aspects of his hearing loss will result in a management plan emphasizing the important role of education in contributing to future academic and economic success.

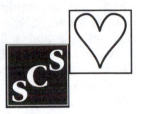

Epilogue

Six years after implantation, Amy Turner is a successful cochlear implant user. Having received the device at age 2 years 7 months, Amy learned to use the new auditory information obtained from the implant to develop speech and spoken language. After her years in the early intervention program, she was placed in a regional preschool program for deaf children close to her home. Amy's speech and language continued to develop as did her auditory skills. Although the educational setting supported the simultaneous use of speech and sign at all times, Amy's functional use of language was primarily through the oral mode. Her family would sign only in situations in which new information was being presented.

Amy made good progress in her self-contained, total communication classroom. She developed early reading and math skills and scored well on tests of academic achievement when compared to her hearing peers. This success led her parents to seek placement for Amy back in her local public school. Supported by the educational consultant from the implant center, the local school designed a program for Amy which placed her in the first grade. With the assistance of a teacher/interpreter (a certified teacher of the deaf who interprets classroom instruction and provides tutorial help) Amy was ranked by her teacher as performing at the top of her class.

Now finishing third grade, Amy is maintaining the social and academic gains accomplished thus far. She has both deaf and normal hearing friends. She appears to be a happy and well-adjusted child with interests and abilities similar to her normal hearing agemates. Amy relies on her implant in everyday communicative exchanges and has achieved open set speech recognition which allows her to use the telephone to speak with family and close friends. Her speech is intelligible even to the naive listener.

Although Amy can function easily in any number of social settings using only oral communication, her educational needs as a deaf child with a cochlear implant cannot be overlooked. Preferential seating, use of caption materials whenever possible, and access to a certified teacher of the deaf are services likely to be required throughout her educational career. In addition, Amy is learning to act as her own advocate by identifying communication situations which are problematic.

The Turners have watched Amy grow and progress and marvel at her journey. They have raised "three Amys" in their lifetime. The first Amy was the normal hearing infant whose early development was unremarkable. Communication with her was effortless and taken for granted. The second Amy appeared after the meningitis and during the period of hearing aid use. This was a time of labored communication with limited responsiveness to speech and environmental sound. Finally, the third Amy is today's Amy. Communication has almost, but not quite, become effortless once again. The Turners themselves now provide support for new families considering the cochlear implant for their child. The cochlear implant may not be for every child, but when candidates are properly selected and carefully monitored, success stories like Amy's are possible.

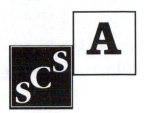

Appendix A
Network of Educators of Children with Cochlear Implants (NECCI)

NETWORK OF EDUCATORS OF CHILDREN WITH COCHLEAR IMPLANTS (NECCI)

Please make your $15.00 check payable to NECCI and return with this form completed to:

NECCI
c/o Cochlear Implant Center
210 East 64th Street
New York, NY 10021
(212) 605-3793 telephone
(212) 838-6239 fax

LAST NAME:_____ **FIRST NAME:**_____

AFFILIATION:_____

ADDRESS:_____

CITY:_____

STATE/PROVINCE:_____

ZIP/POSTAL CODE:_____

COUNTRY:_____

TELEPHONE:_____

FAX NUMBER:_____

E MAIL ADDRESS:_____

DESCRIPTION: Educator   Audiologist   Administrator
(circle all that apply)   Teacher Prep   Parent   AV Therapist
                     Speech Language Pathologist
                     Other (please specify)_____

LIST IN DIRECTORY: circle one please   yes   no

Signature:_____ date_____

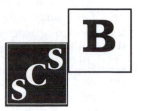

Appendix B
Sample Letter to Parents Regarding Hospital Stay

Dear Parents,

The arrangements for your child's cochlear implant surgery have been made and there are some details regarding his/her hospital stay which are important for you to know.

You should arrive at the hospital at 6:00 AM on the day of surgery, to register, obtain a room and change into the hospital issued pajamas. Your child should not have had anything to eat or drink since midnight the previous day. One of the audiologists from the Implant Center will meet you in your room to accompany your child to the operating suite. If your child has a "security blanket," stuffed animal, or special toy which helps relax him/her, it may be brought into surgery. It will be returned to you after the procedure is completed. The audiologist will remain with your child while he/she is awake and will return to test the device once it has been implanted.

When your child returns to the room following surgery, there will be a fairly large bandage on his/her head and a small plastic tubing (drain) exiting from the incision. On the average, the children sleep through most of the remaining portion of the day. One parent is permitted to remain in the room overnight and a reclining chair will be provided for sleeping. Arrangements can be made for closed caption television and for any other assistive devices you might require.

Most children prefer to change into their own pajamas the day after surgery. You should bring shirts which button or snap so that nothing tight goes over the child's head. This also applies to the clothing for the trip home. T-shirts, turtlenecks, or sweatshirts should be avoided because it will be difficult to pull them over the bandage.

The nurses at our facility are familiar with the follow-up procedures for cochlear implants. If your child is uncomfortable or you have any questions regarding any immediate medical issues, you should direct any of these to them. They are able to contact Dr. (Name of implanting surgeon) or any of the other on-call physicians.

If you have any additional questions, please feel free to contact me at (XXX) XXX-XXXX.

Sincerely,

Director
Cochlear Implant Center

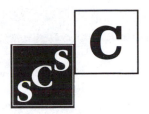

Appendix C
Parents' Dictionary
Nucleus 22
Channel Implant

In anticipation of the initial hook up of your child's cochlear implant there are a few terms and concepts that we believe will be helpful for you to understand prior to the appointment.

Electrode Array   This is made up of 22 electrode bands and 10 retaining rings. The array is designed with the low numbered electrodes (#1) stimulating the high frequency area of the cochlea and the high numbered electrodes (#22) stimulating the low frequency area of the cochlea.

Threshold Level   The level at which the patient first identifies sound sensation and the lowest level at which the child hears the stimulus every time it is presented. These levels are not related to decibels and are commonly called T-Levels.

Comfort Level   This is the maximum level for a series of pulses that does not produce an uncomfortable loudness sensation for the implant user. These levels are not related to decibels and are commonly called C-Levels.

Map/Mapping The setting of the speech processor according to an individual's measured threshold and comfort levels and subjective responses to sound.

Dynamic Range The number of units between the threshold and comfort levels.

Active Electrode The half of the electrode pair that begins stimulation.

Indifferent Electrode The half of the electrode pair that acts as the ground for the electric current.

Stimulation Mode This determines how much of the electrode array is stimulated each time. When more current is required to obtain T and C levels an increase in the area of stimulation will occur by changing the stimulation mode.

Common Ground (CG)	This stimulation mode allows for the use of all 22 electrodes. When one electrode is chosen as the active electrode all of the remaining electrodes are connected together and become the indifferent electrode.
Bipolar (BP)	The stimulation mode in which the active and indifferent electrodes are beside each other (i.e., #22 = indifferent, #21 = active).
Bipolar + 1 (BP+1)	The stimulation mode in which there is one electrode in between the active and indifferent electrodes (i.e., #22 = indifferent, #20 = active).
Bipolar + 2 (BP+2)	The stimulation mode in which there are two electrodes in between the active and indifferent electrodes (i.e., #22 = indifferent, #19 = active).
Bipolar + 3 (BP+3)	The stimulation mode in which there are three electrodes in between the active and indifferent electrodes (i.e., #22 = indifferent, #18 = active).

Strategy This determines how the information is sent through the cochlear implant. The two most common strategies used are called Multipeak (**MPEAK**) and Spectral Peak (**SPEAK**).

SPEAK   This strategy is the most recently developed one from the manufacturer of this device and can only be programmed if your child has a *Spectra* speech processor. It identifies the six most prominent peaks of the incoming signal and presents the information to electrodes which correspond to the frequency content of the signal.

MPEAK   This strategy is the most commonly used in the *MSP* speech processor. It identifies four different parts of the speech signal (known as speech features) and assigns each part to a different electrode.

Stimulation Units/Current Level   The level of the signal presented through the speech processor. These are the units of current which are delivered through the implant; **decibels are not used** since the signal is an electrical and not acoustical one.

Sensitivity Control   The dial on top of the processor which sets the responsiveness of the microphone to the sound source. With a low sensitivity setting the sound source must be very close to the microphone. With a high sensitivity setting, the sound source can be further from the microphone.

Transmitter Cord   The short cord which connects the microphone to the transmitter coil.

Processor Cord   The long cord which connects the microphone to the speech processor. The dot on the cord must match the dot on the microphone for the system to work correctly.

External Input of Processor   A location on the speech processor in which external devices (telephone, walkman, etc.) can be attached to the speech processor. This area should be kept covered when not in use and cleaned periodically to remove the dust and dirt which accumulates.

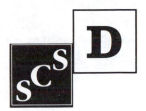

Appendix D
Parents' Dictionary
Clarion Multi
Strategy System

In anticipation of the initial hook up of your child's cochlear implant there are a few terms and concepts that we believe will be helpful for you to understand prior to the appointment.

Electrode Array   This electrode array is made up of 16 ball electrodes. These electrodes are placed in pairs and are labelled as being medial or lateral. The array is numbered with the low numbered electrodes (#1) stimulating the low frequency area of the cochlea and the high numbered electrodes stimulating the high frequency area of the cochlea.

Threshold Level   The level at which the patient first identifies sound sensation and the lowest level at which the child hears the stimulus every time it is presented. These levels are not related to decibels and are commonly called T-Levels.

Most Comfortable Level   This is the maximum level for a series of pulses which does not produce an uncomfortable loudness sensation for the implant user. These levels are not related to decibels and are commonly called M-Levels.

Program   The setting of the speech processor according to an individual's measured threshold and comfort levels and subjective responses to sound.

Dynamic Range   The number of units between the threshold and comfort levels.

Active Electrode   The half of the electrode pair that begins stimulation.

Indifferent Electrode   The half of the electrode pair that acts as the ground for the electric current.

Stimulation Mode   This determines how much of the electrode array is stimulated each time. When more current is required to obtain T and M levels, an increase in the area of stimulation will occur by changing the stimulation mode. The Clarion can be programmed in a Bipolar mode or in a Monopolar mode.

Bipolar Mode   In a bipolar mode the current flows between two electrodes which are situated close to one another. The distance between the two electrodes is very small.

Monopolar Mode   In a monopolar mode, the current flows between an electrode and an area much further away. The distance between these two areas is much greater.

Strategy   The process used to transform the incoming speech signal into a particular pattern of electrical stimulation. The Clarion device can be programmed using a Compressed Analog (**CA**) or Continuous Interleaved Sampling (**CIS**) strategy.

>   **CA**   This strategy uses a series of filters which are assigned to different frequencies. The signal is delivered to the appropriate filters depending on the frequency of the incoming sound. Each of these filters is assigned to a pair of electrodes which is stimulated when the signal is sent through the speech processor.

>   **CIS**   This strategy sends the speech signal to the electrodes through a series of very rapid pulses.

Stimulation Units/Current Level   The level of the signal presented through the speech processor. These are the units of current which are delivered through the implant; **decibels are not used** because the signal is an electrical and not acoustical one.

Sensitivity Control   The dial on top of the processor which sets the responsiveness of the microphone to the sound source. With a low sensitivity setting, the sound source must be very close to the microphone. With a high sensitivity setting, the sound source can be further from the microphone.

Volume Control   The dial on the top of the processor which controls the loudness of the sound transmitted to the headset.

Processor Cord   The long cord which connects the speech processor to the headpiece.

Mic Input of Processor   A location on the speech processor in which external devices (telephone, walkman, etc.) can be attached to speech processor. This area should be kept covered when not in use and cleaned periodically to remove the dust and dirt which accumulates.

Program Selector   A dial on the top of the processor which is numbered from 1–3. This selects the speech processing strategy in use by the patient.

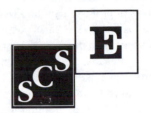

Appendix E
Letter Regarding
Initial Stimulation

Dear Parents,

We have scheduled an appointment for (child's name) to come to the Cochlear Implant Center at (Institution Name) for his/her initial "tune-up"on (Date) at (Time) and on (Date) at (Time). At that time (Child's Name) will receive the external equipment for his/her cochlear implant and the device will be programmed. This process takes place over the course of two days.

On the first day we will fit him/her with all of the external equipment (microphone, transmitter, and speech processor), set as many electrodes as possible, and create a unique program known as a "map" for your child. The first day's session will last approximately five hours. We have enclosed a Parents' Dictionary of Terms which we will be using throughout the tune-up process. We would urge you to read it carefully so as to familiarize yourself with much of the new language which is particular to the cochlear implant.

The second day's session will last between 3 and 5 hours depending on your child. The program will be fine-tuned and we will begin some basic auditory lessons. In addition to fine tuning the program, we will train you in how to troubleshoot the equipment as well as how to manage the daily wear and care of the implant. We will also review with you the strategies which will help you foster good listening skills with your child at home. If there are any other family members or professionals who would be interested in attending these sessions, please let us know as soon as possible. You should be aware, however, that too many observers in the room during the tune-up process is often disruptive.

Because you will be returning home with a substantial amount of equipment in boxes, we suggest that you bring a large shopping bag with you. Because there are a variety of ways to wear the processor, we suggest that your child wear clothing which has a belt or a shirt with a pocket. Children's pouches have a harness attachment which can be worn under their clothing or, if you/they prefer, you may bring a bicycle or "fanny" pouch.

On the average, reprogramming is necessary at one, three, and six months from the date of initial stimulation. Your child will be seen every six months thereafter. Very young children (ages 2–4 years) are seen every two weeks for the first two months. (Remember, however, there may be exceptions to this schedule.) The exact number of visits will depend on your child's responses to the tune-up process.

The cost of the initial tune-up is $XXX.XX. Follow-up visits are billed at the rate of $XXX.XX per hour. A payment schedule for the initial stimulation and the follow-up visits is listed below. Payment is due at the time the service is rendered. Major credit cards are accepted. The paid receipt can be attached to the necessary insurance papers for reimbursement from your insurance company.

The following fee schedule has been devised so that we can secure payment in a timely fashion without creating an unnecessary financial burden to the family.

	Billed	**Must Pay**
Initial tune-up	$XXX.XX	$XXX.XX
1 month retune	$XXX.XX	$XXX.XX
3 month retune	$XXX.XX	$XXX.XX
6 month retune	$XXX.XX	$XXX.XX

If you have any questions, please call the office at (XXX) XXX-XXXX.

Sincerely,

Director
Cochlear Implant Center

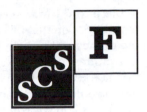

Appendix F
Nucleus 22 Channel
Cochlear Implant System
Troubleshooting Guide

The following is the recommended sequence of tests which should be performed when there is a suspected problem with the implant. These problems include: *no sound heard by the user, distorted sounds, or background noises.* If the sequence is followed appropriately, you should be able to identify the problem.

Step 1.
Replace battery with a fully charged battery or a new alkaline AA battery. Test the unit by setting the selector switch to "T." The red "M" light should be steady and bright. If the unit fails to work after replacing the batteries proceed to the next step.

Step 2.
Clean battery contacts with alcohol. Retest processor as noted above. If the unit fails to work, proceed to the next step.

Step 3.

Replace cord from processor to microphone (long cord). Make certain that the dot on the cord and the dot on the microphone match up. Test the unit by setting selector switch to "N," the "on" position. Place the transmitter coil on the external portion of the speech processor on the side marked with the name "Cochlear." When this is done, the red "C" light should be shimmering (it may not be very bright or completely steady). If you speak into the microphone the "M" light will go on and off along with your voice. If the unit still fails to work, proceed to the next step.

Step 4.

Replace the cord from the transmitter to the microphone (short cord). (You should check to insure that the two prongs on the short cord are not green from mildew. A toothbrush dipped in alcohol can usually alleviate this problem). Test the unit in the manner noted in Step 3. If the unit fails to work, proceed to the next step.

Step 5.

Plug the hand-held (auxiliary) microphone into the external jack on top of the processor. Speak into the microphone. The red "M" light should go on and off with speech. If the unit fails to work, proceed to the next step.

Step 6.

If you have followed all of the steps and your child still hears nothing and the lights on the processor are not lighting appropriately, you must call your local Cochlear Implant Center to arrange for a new processor.

After trying the above remedies, if the problem persists, contact the appropriate person for support.

Cochlear Corporation
61 Inverness Drive, Suite 200
Englewood, CO 80112
(800) 523-5798 (Voice/TDD)

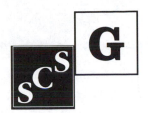

Appendix G
Clarion Multistrategy Cochlear Implant System Troubleshooting Guide

Problem	Solution
No Sound Heard: No Response from User	While watching the LED light on the Speech Processor (SP), turn the SP off and then back on to position 1. If you see: *No light*, replace the Clarion battery pack with another fully charged battery pack or 3 AA size Alkaline batteries. *1 to 4 quick blinks and then 3 long blinks*, replace the cable. *1 to 4 quick blinks and then 1 long blink and **no sound** is heard*, replace the headpiece. *(continued)*

	Note: If a headpiece is not available, use an auxiliary microphone *1 to 4 quick blinks and then 1 long blink,* this means that the system is functioning normally and sounds should be heard.
User Hears Static Sounds	Replace the cable
User Hears Muffled or Distorted Sound	Remove any material which may be covering the headpiece microphone opening.
Headpiece or Speech Processor Gets Wet	Remove the battery pack from the Speech processor and place the entire unit in a Dri-Aid pack. Contact the cochlear implant facility immediately. DO NOT ATTEMPT TO CLEAN OR DRY UNIT. DO NOT USE A HAIR DRYER OR OTHER ELECTRICAL APPLIANCE TO DRY THE UNIT.
Check the Battery Status	While watching the LED light on the Speech Processor (SP), turn the SP off and then back to position 1. If you see: *3 to 4 quick blinks,* this indicates that the battery is fully charged and should last about 8 hours. *2 to 3 quick blinks,* this indicates that the battery should last about 4–5 hours. <div align="right">*(continued)*</div>

	1 quick blink, this indicates that the battery should last about 1 hour.
Speech Processor, Headpiece, or Cable needs to be Cleaned	Clean each component with a soft dry or lightly dampened cloth. Never use solvents or abrasive cleaners which might damage the finish of the component.

After trying the above remedies, if the problem persists, contact the appropriate person for support.

Advanced Bionics Corporation
Clarion Cochlear Implant System
12740 San Fernando Road
Sylmar, CA 91342-3700
(800) 678-2575 (Voice)
(800) 678-3575 (TDD)

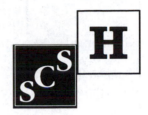

Appendix H
Closed Set Tests of
Speech Perception

Test Name	Type	Stimulus Materials	Percent Chance
Glendonald Auditory Screening Procedure (GASP)	Stress	Mono, Spondee, Trochee, 3-syllable	25
	Word	3 words in each category	33
Monosyllable-Trochee-Spondee Test (MTS)	Stress	Monosyllabic, Spondee, Trochee	33
	Word	4 words in each stress category	25
Early Speech Perception Test (ESP)	Pattern Perception	3 words in each category: monosyllable, spondee, trochee, 3-syllable	25
	Spondee Identification	12 spondaic words	8
	Monosyllable Identification	12 monosyllabic words	8
Early Speech Perception Test (ESP) Low Verbal Version	Pattern Perception	4 toys: monosyllable, spondee, trochee, 3-syllable	25
	Spondee Identification	4 spondees	25
	Monosyllable Identification	4 monosyllables	25

Test Name	Type	Stimulus Materials	Percent Chance
Northwestern University Children's Perception of Speech (NU-Chips)	Word	Single syllable words 4 lists of 50 words	25
Word Intelligibility by Picture Inventory (WIPI)	Word	Single syllable words 4 lists of 25 words	17
Minimal Pairs	Word	Pairs of monosyllable words that differ in voicing, manner, place, vowel height, and vowel place	40 overall score 8 each contrast

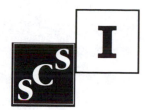

Appendix I
Open Set Tests of Speech Perception

Test Name	Type	Stimulus Materials
Phonetically Balanced Kindergarten Word List (PBK)	Word	Monosyllable words 2 lists of 50
City University of New York Sentences (CUNY Sentences)	Key word	60 blocks of 12 sentences in each block with a total of 102 words per sentence

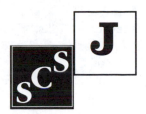

Appendix J
Mainstream Checklist

**Checklist for Observing Classroom Participation
of Hearing-Impaired Student**

Mary Ellen Nevins and Patricia M. Chute

Cochlear Implant Center
Manhattan Eye, Ear and Throat Hospital
210 East 64th Street
New York, NY 10021

Date:_____   Student:_____
Age of Student:_____   Grade Level:_____

The Classroom

Teacher/
Class Observed: _____ Length of Observation:_____
Class Size: _____Diagram of Physical Arrangement
(*student's location)

Number of
Teachers/Adults:_____

Style of
Presentation: _ Teacher Directed _ Guest Speaker _ Student Speaker

          _ Group Discussion   _ Co-op. Learning

Student Performance

1. General response to environmental sounds:

1	2	3	4
Appears unaware of environmental sounds	Responds to some sounds	Looks for source of sound	Appears to recognize familiar sounds

List some of these sounds:

_____

2. General response to speech:

1	2	3	4	5
No apparent response to speech	Occasional response to speech	Must be prompted to listen	Understands when able to look and listen	Understands speech through hearing alone

3. Knowledge of classroom routines; handling transitions:

1	2	3	4
Appears unaware of routine/does not makes transitions	Makes transitions with adult assistance	Makes transition by observing others	Aware of routine/ makes transitions independently

4. Following directions:

1	2	3
Does not follow directions	Follows with help	Follows independently

5. Attention to classroom instruction:

1	2	3	4	5
Disengaged	Attends less than 25% of time	Attends 50% of time	Attends 75% of time	Attends 100% of time

6. Comprehension of classroom instruction:

1	2	3	4
Does not comprehend	Appears to understand information that is familiar/highly structured	Appears to understand information that is new or less structured	Appears to understand everything

Provide a narrative of how the child handled a typical instructional session; cite indicators that the student was using his hearing

_____

_____

7. Typical behavior when content was not understood:

1	2	3	4	5
Drops out/ engages in irrelevant activity	Facial cues indicate lack of under- standing	Looks to another student for assistance	Asks for assistance from teacher	Indicates specifically content not understood

Outline context, record question and teacher response (include role of interpreter in this exchange) in one child-teacher exchange

8. Typical recitation behavior

1	2	3	4
Disengaged	Does not respond when called	Answers when called upon	Volunteers

Provide a narrative of a typical interaction

9a. Student's response and comments in lecture/teacher directed activities

1	2	3	4	5
None made	Inappropriate to the topic	Incorrect but appropriate	Correct and appropriate	Enriching to the discussion

Cite typical examples

9b. Student's responses and comments in group discussion

1	2	3	4	5
Disengaged	Attentive initially; gives up	Attentive; does not comment	Attentive; comments inappropriately	Attentive and comments appropriately

Provide context in which this happens

_____

_____

10. Typical interactions with peers (Mark highest level)

Receptive

1	2	3	4
Not approached	Approached/ does not respond	Approached/ responds inappropriately	Approached/ responds appropriately

Record frequency of this behavior; provide examples if possible

_____

_____

Expressive

	1	2	3
	Does not initiate	Initiates inappropriately	Initiates appropriately

Record frequency of this behavior; provide examples if possible

_____

_____

Is this child's behavior during observation typical of his overall performance?

_____

_____

Additional Comments:_____

_____

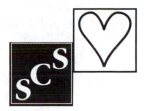

References

Allen, T. E. (1986). Patterns of academic achievement among hearing-impaired students: 1974–1983. In A. Shildroth & M. Karchmer (Eds.), *Deaf children in America*. San Diego: College-Hill Press.

Allen, T., & Osborn, T. (1984). Academic integration of hearing-impaired students: Demographic, handicapping and achievement factors. *American Annals of the Deaf, 129*, 100–113.

Antia, S. D. (1982). Social interactions of partially mainstreamed hearing-impaired children. *American Annals of the Deaf, 127*, 18–25.

Bellman, S. (1994, May). *Assessing multiply-handicapped children for cochlear implantation*. Paper presented at the meeting of the European Symposium on Paediatric Cochlear Implantation, Montpelier, France.

Berg, F. (1987). *Facilitating classroom listening: A handbook for teachers of normal and hard of hearing children*. Boston: College-Hill Press/Little, Brown.

Berliner, K. I., & Eisenberg, L. S. (1985). Methods and issues in the cochlear implantation of children: An overview. *Ear and Hearing, 6*(Suppl.), 6S–13S.

Bilger, R. C., Black, F. O., Hopkinson, N. T., Myers, E. N., Payne, J. L., Stenson, N. R., Vega, A., & Wolf, R. V. (1977). Evaluation of subjects presently fitted with implanted auditory prostheses. *Annals of Otology Rhinology and Laryngology. 86*(Suppl.), 3–10.

Boothroyd, A. (1976). *Influence of residual hearing on speech perception and speech production by hearing-impaired children*. Paper presented at the annual convention of the American Speech Language and Hearing Association, Houston, TX.

Boothroyd, A. (1982). *Hearing impairments in young children.* Englewood Cliffs, NJ: Prentice Hall.

Boothroyd, A. (1993). Profound deafness. In R. S. Tyler (Ed.), *Cochlear implants: Audiological foundations* (pp. 1–33). San Diego: Singular Publishing.

Brackett, D., & Zara, C. V. (1994, November). *Cochlear implants and the borderline candidate: Making the decision.* Paper presented at the annual convention of the American Speech-Language Hearing Assoication, New Orleans, LA.

Brookhauser, P. E., & Moeller, M. P. (1986). Choosing the appropriate habilitative track for the newly identified hearing-impaired child. *Annals of Otology,Rhinology, and Laryngology, 95,* 51–59.

Calvert, D. R., & Silverman, S. R. (1983). *Speech and deafness.* (Revised). Washington, DC: A. G. Bell Association for the Deaf.

Carle, E. (1969). *The very hungry caterpillar.* Scranton: Collins World.

Castle, D. L. (1988). *Telephone strategies: A technical and practical guide for hard-of-hearing people.* Bethesda, MD: Self Help for Hard of Hearing People, Inc.

Chute, P. M. (1992). The cluster phenomenon. *Necci News, 2*(2), 4.

Chute, P. M. (1993). Cochlear implants in adolescents. In B. Fraysse & O. Deguine (Eds.), *Cochlear implants: New perspectives* (pp. 210–215). Basel: Karger.

Chute, P. M., & Nevins, M.E. (1994, May). *Educational placements of children with multichannel cochlear implants.* Paper presented at the meeting of the European Symposium on Paediatric Cochlear Implantation, Montpelier, France.

Chute, P. M., & Nevins, M. E. (1995). Cochlear implants in people who are deaf/blind. *Journal of Visual Impairment and Blindness, 89,* 297–300.

Clark, G. M. (1987). The University of Melbourne-Nucleus multi-electrode cochlear implant. *Advances in Oto-Rhino-Laryngology, 38,* 124–126.

Clark, G. M., Cohen, N. L., & Sheppard, R. K. (1991). Surgical and safety considerations in multi channel cochlear implants in children. *Ear and Hearing, 12,* 15S–24S.

Cochlear Corporation. (1993). Mini system 22 cochlear implant reliability report. *Clinical Bulletin.* (pp.1–6) Englewood, CO: Cochlear Corporation.

Cochlear Corporation. (1994). *Technical reference manual* (p. 119). Englewood, CO: Cochlear Corporation.

Cowan, R. S. C., Brown, C., Whitford, L. A., Galvin, K. L., Sarant, J. Z., Barker, E. J., Shaw, S., King, A., Skok, M., Seligman, P. M., Dowell, R. C., Gibson, W. P. R., & Clark, G. (1994, October). *Speech perception in children using the advanced SPEAK speech processing strategy.* Paper presented at the meeting of the International Cochlear Implant, Speech and Hearing Symposium, Melbourne, Australia.

Craig, W., & Craig H. (1975). (Eds.) Directory of services for the Deaf, *American Annals of the Deaf, 120,* 118.

DeFillipo, C., & Scott, B. (1978). A method for training and evaluating the reception of ongoing speech. *Journal of the Acoustical Society of America, 63*(4), 1186–1192.

Djourno, A., & Eyries, C. (1957). Prosthese auditive par excitation electrique a sistance du nerf sensoriel a l'aide d'un bobinage inclus a demeure. *Presse Med, 35,* 14–17.

Dowell, R. C., Mecklenburg, D. J., & Clark, G. M. (1986). Speech recognition for 40 patients receiving multichannel cochlear implants. *Archives of Otolaryngology, 112*, 1054–1059.

Dowell, R. C., Seligman, P. M., Blamey, P. J., & Clark, G. M. (1987). Evaluation of a two-formant speech processing strategy for a multichannel cochlear prosthesis. *Annals of Otology, Rhinology and Laryngology, 96*(Suppl. 128), 132–134.

Economou, A., Tartter, V. C., Chute, P. M., & Hellman, S. A. (1992). Speech changes following reimplantation from a single-channel to a multichannel cochlear implant. *Journal of the Acoustical Society of America, 92*(3), 1310–1323.

Eilers, R. E., Vergara, K. C., Cobo-Lewis, A., & Oller, D. K. (1994). *Performance of deaf children using tactile aids and cochlear implants.* Paper presented at the annual American Speech-Language Hearing Association, New Orleans, LA.

Elliot, L., & Katz, D. (1980). *Development of a new children's test of speech discrimination.* St. Louis, MO: Auditec.

Erber, N. P. (1982). *Auditory training.* Washington, DC: A. G. Bell Association for the Deaf.

Erber, N. P., & Alencewicz, C. (1976). Audiologic evaluation of deaf children. *Journal of Speech and Hearing Disorders, 41*, 256–267.

Evans, J. W. (1989). Thoughts on the psychosocial implications of cochlear implantation in children. In E. Owens & D. Kessler (Eds.), *Cochlear implants in young deaf children,* Boston: College-Hill Press.

Firszt, J., Reeder, R., & Novak, M. (in press). Multichannel cochlear implantation with inner ear malformation: Case report of performance and management. *The Journal of the American Academy of Audiology.*

Gantz, B. J., McCabe, B. F., & Tyler, R. S. (1988). Use of multichannel cochlear implants in obstructed and obliterated cochleas. *Otolaryngology Head and Neck Surgery 98*, 72–81.

Gantz, B. J., Tyler, R. S., Woodworth, G. G., Tye-Murray, N., & Fryauf-Bertschy, H. (1994). Results of multichannel cochlear implants in congenital and acquired prelingual deafness in children: Five-year follow up. *American Journal of Otology, 15*(Suppl.), 107.

Gantz, B. J., Tyler, R. S., Lowder, M. W., & Woodworth, G. G. (1995). *Preliminary results with three different multichannel cochlear implant systems in postlingually deafened adults.* Paper presented at the meeting of the International Cochlear Implant, Speech and Hearing Symposium, Melbourne, Australia.

Geers, A. E., & Moog, J. S. (1987). Predicting spoken language acquisition in profoundly deaf children. *Journal of Speech and Hearing Disorders, 52*(1), 84–94.

Geers, A. E., & Moog, J. S. (1991). Evaluating the benefits of cochlear implants in an educational setting. *The American Journal of Otology, 12*(Suppl.), 116–125.

Geier, L., Gilden, J., Luetje, C.M., & Maddox, H. E. III. (1993). Delayed perception of cochlear implant stimulation in children with postmeningitic ossified cochleae. *American Journal of Otology, 14*, 556–561.

Good, T. L., & Brophy, J. E. (1994). *Looking in classrooms.* New York: Harper & Row.

Haskins, H. A. (1949). *A phonetically balanced test of speech discrimination for children.* Unpublished masters thesis, Northwestern University, Evanston, IL.

Hellman, S. A., Chute, P. M., Kretschmer, R. E., Nevins, M. E., Parisier, S.C., & Thurston, L. C. (1991). The development of a children's implant profile. *American Annals of the Deaf, 136*, 77–81.

Hodges, A. V., Ruth, R. A., Thomas, J. F., & Blincoe, C. S., (1991, November). *Electrically evoked ABRs and ARs in cochlear implant users.* Paper presented at the meeting of the American Speech-Language-Hearing Association Convention, Atlanta, GA.

House, W. F., & Berliner, K. (1991) Cochlear implants: From idea to clinical practice. In H. Cooper (Ed.), *Cochlear implants: A practical guide* (pp. 9–33). San Diego: Singular Publishing.

House, W. F., & Urban, J. (1973). Long-term results of electrode implantation and electronic stimulation of the cochlea in man. *Annals of Otology, Rhinology and Laryngology, 82*, 504–517.

Hudgins, C. V., & Numbers, F. C. (1942). An investigation of intelligibility of the speech of the deaf. *Genetic Psychology Monographs, 25*, 289–392.

Johnson, R. E., Liddell, S. K., & Erting, C. J. (1989). *Unlocking the curriculum: Principles for achieving access in deaf education* (working paper, pp. 89-93). Washington, DC: Gallaudet Research Institute.

Kemink, J. L., Zimmerman-Phillips, S., Kileny, P. R., Firszt, J. B., & Novak, M. A. (1992). Auditory performance of children with cochlear ossification and partial implant insertion. *Laryngoscope, 102*, 1001–1005.

Kessler, D. K., Zilberman, Y., Roff, D., & Loeb, G. E. (1994, October). *Distribution of speech recognition results with the Clarion cochlear prosthesis.* Paper presented at the meeting of the International Cochlear Implant, Speech and Hearing Symposium, Melbourne, Australia.

Kirk, K. I., Sehgal, M., & Miyamoto, R. T. (in press). Speech perception performance of Nucleus multichannel cochlear implant users with partial electrode insertions. *Ear and Hearing.*

Knoff, H. M. (1983). Personality assessment in the schools: Issues and procedures for school psychologists. *School Psychology Review, 12*, 391–398.

Knoff, H. M. (1987). Assessing adolescent identity, self-concept, and self-esteem. In R. G. Harrington (Ed.), *Testing adolescents: A reference guide for comprehensive psychological assessments* (pp. 51–81). St. Louis: Westport Publishers.

Lane, H. (1992). *The mask of benevolence.* New York: Alfred A. Knopf.

Lesinski, A., Hartrampf, R., Dahm, M. C., Bertram, B., Straub-Schier, A., & Lenarz, T. (1994, October). *Cochlear implantation in a population of multihandicapped children.* Paper presented at the meeting of the International Cochlear Implant, Speech and Hearing Symposium, Melbourne, Australia.

Ling, D. (1976). *Speech and the hearing-impaired child: Theory and practice.* Washington, DC: A. G. Bell Association for the Deaf.

Ling, D. (1986). Devices and procedures for auditory learning. *The Volta Review, 88*, 19–28.

Manning, D. (1990). Supportive mainstreaming from a residential school. In M. Ross (Ed.), *Hearing-impaired children in the mainstream.* Parkton, MD: York Press.

Manolson, A. (1985). *It takes two to talk.* Toronto: Ontario Institute for Studies in Education.

Matkin, N., Hook, P., & Hixson, P. (1979). A multidisciplinary approach to evaluation of hearing-impaired children. *Audiology: A Journal of Continuing Education.*

McKay, C. M., & McDermott, H. J. (1991). Speech perception ability of adults with multiple-channel cochlear implants, using the spectral maxima sound processor. *Journal of the Acoustical Society of America, 89*(Suppl. 1), 19–59.

Medwetsky, L. (1994). Educational audiology. In J. Katz (Ed.), *Handbook of clinical audiology* (pp. 503–520). Baltimore: Wilkins & Wilkins.

Mertens, D. M. (1989). Social experiences of hearing-impaired high school youth. *American Annals of the Deaf, 134,* 15–19.

Mischook, M., & Cole, E. (1986). Auditory learning and teaching of hearing-impaired infants. *The Volta Review, 88,* 67–81.

Moog, J. S., & Geers, A. E. (1990). *Early Speech Perception Test.* St. Louis, MO: Central Institute for the Deaf.

Moores, D. (1987). *Educating the deaf.* Boston: Houghton Mifflin.

Myres, W., & Kessler, K. (1992). Understanding the Map. Necci News, 3, 1.

National Association of the Deaf. (1991). NAD position paper on cochlear implants. NAD Broadcaster. Cited in *NECCI News* 2, 1.

Nevins, M. E. (1986). *Multidisciplinary assessment of the hearing-impaired child.* Panel participant at the Texas Speech/Language and Hearing Association Annual Convention. Austin, Texas.

Nevins, M. E. (1994). Yearly transitions pose challenges to school personnel. *Necci News, 5,* 1.

Nevins, M. E., & Chute, P. M. (1994, October). *The success of children with cochlear implants in mainstream educational settings.* Paper presented at the meeting of the International Cochlear Implant, Speech and Hearing Symposium, Melbourne, Australia.

Nevins, M. E., Kretschmer, R. E. Chute, P. M., Hellman, S. A., & Parisier, S.C. (1991). The role of an educational consultant in a pediatric cochlear implant program. *The Volta Review, 93,* 197–204.

Novak, M., Firszt, J. B., Brown, C., & Reeder, R. (1990). *Cochlear implantation in severe cochlear deformities.* Paper presented at the Second International Cochlear Implant Symposium, Iowa.

Osberger, M. J., Chute, P. M., Pope, M., Kessler, K. S., Carotta, C. C., Firszt, J., & Zimmerman-Philips, S. (1991a). Pediatric cochlear implant candidacy issues. *The American Journal of Otology, 12*(Suppl.), 80–88.

Osberger, M. J., Miyamoto, R. T., Zimmerman-Phillips, S., Kemink, J. L., Stroer, B. S., Firszt, J. B., & Novak, M. A. (1991b). Independent evaluation of the speech perception abilities of children with the Nucleus 22-Channel cochlear implant system. *Ear and Hearing, 12*(Suppl. 4), 66S–80S.

Osberger, M. J., Robbins, A. M., Miyamoto, R. T., Berry, S. W., Myres, W. A., Kessler, K. S., & Pope, M. L. (1991c). Speech perception abilities of children with cochlear implants, tactile aids, or hearing aids. *The American Journal of Otology, 12*(Suppl.), 105–115.

Osberger, M. J., Robbins, A. M., Todd, S. L., & Riley, A.I. (1994). Speech intelligibility of children with cochlear implants. *Volta Review, 96*, 169–180.

Parisier, S. C., & Chute, P. M. (1993). Multichannel implants in postmeningitic ossified cochleas. In B. Fraysse & O. Deguine (Eds.), *Cochlear implants: New perspectives* (pp. 49–58). Basel: Karger.

Parisier, S. C., & Chute, P. M. (1994, May). *Speech production changes in children using multichannel cochlear implants.* Paper presented at the meeting of the European Symposium on Paediatric Cochlear Implantation, Montpelier, France.

Parisier, S. C., Chute, P. M., & Nevins, M. E. (1994). Pediatric cochlear implants: Surgical and rehabilitative issues. In F. E. Lucente (Ed.), *Highlights of the instructional courses* (pp. 145–154). St. Louis: Mosby.

Paterson, M. (1986). Maximizing the use of residual hearing with school-aged hearing-impaired students—A perspective. *The Volta Review, 88*, 93–105.

Patrick, J. F., & Clark, G. M. (1991). The Nucleus 22-channel cochlear implant system. *Ear and Hearing, 12*(Suppl. 1), 3S–9S.

Paul, P., & Quigley, S. (1984). *Language and deafness.* San Diego: College-Hill Press.

Perigoe, C. B. (1992). Strategies for the remediation of speech of hearing-impaired children. In R. Stoker & D. Ling (Eds.), Speech production in hearing impaired children and youth. *The Volta Review, 94*, 95–118.

Pflaster, G. (1980). A factor analysis of variables related to academic performance of hearing-impaired children in regular classes. *The Volta Review, 82*, 71–84.

Plant, G. (1989). *Tactaid II training program.* Sydney, Australia: National Acoustics Laboratories.

Robbins, A. M. (1994, February). *A critical evaluation of rehabilitation techniques.* Paper presented at the 5th Symposium on Cochlear Implants in Children, New York, NY.

Ross, M., Brackett, D., & Maxon, A. (1991). *Assessment and management of mainstreamed hearing-impaired children.* Austin: Pro-Ed.

Ross, M., & Lerman, J. (1971). *Word intelligibility by picture identification.* Pittsburgh: Stanwix House, Inc.

Sarant, J. Z., Cowan, R. S. C., Blamey, P. J., Galvin, K. L., & Clark, G. M. (1994). Cochlear implants for congenitally deaf adolescents: Is open-set speech perception a realistic expectation? *Ear and Hearing, 15*(5), 400–403.

Schwartz, S. (1987). *Choices in deafness.* Rockville, MD: Woodbine House.

Skinner, M. W. (1994, February). *The borderline child.* Paper presented at the meeting of the 5th Symposium on Cochlear Implants in Children, New York, NY.

Skinner, M. W., Forakis, M., Holden, L. K., & Holden, T. A. (1994, October). *Comparison of postlinguistically deaf adults identification of vowels and consonants with SPEAK and MPEAK speech processing strategies of the Nucleus cochlear implant system.* Paper presented at the meeting of the International Cochlear Implant Speech and Hearing Symposium, Melbourne, Australia.

Skinner, M. W., Holden, L. K., Holden, T. A., Dowell, R. C., Seligman, P. M., Brimacombe, J. A., & Beiter, A. L. (1991). Performance of postlinguistically deaf adults with the Wearable Speech Processor (WSP III) and Mini Speech Processor (MSP) of the Nucleus multi-electrode cochlear implant. *Ear and Hearing, 12,* 3–22.

Spivak, L. G., & Chute, P. M. (1994). The relationship between electrical acoustic reflex thresholds and behavioral comfort levels in children and adult cochlear implant patients. *Ear and Hearing, 15,* 184–192.

Spragins, A. B. (1987). Consideration in assessing the psychological adjustment of handicapped adolescents. In R. G. Harrington (Ed.), *Testing adolescents: A reference guide for comprehensive psychological assessments* (pp. 51–81). St. Louis: Westport Publishers.

Staller, S. J., Beiter, A. L., & Brimacombe, J. A. (1994). Use of the Nucleus 22 channel cochlear implant system with children. *Volta Review, 96,* 15–40.

Staller, S. J., Dowell, R. C., Beiter, A. L., & Brimacombe, J. A. (1991). Perceptual abilities of children with the Nucleus 22-channel cochlear implant. *Ear and Hearing, 12*(4), 34S–47S.

Thielemeir, M. (1985). Status and results of the House Ear Institute cochlear implant project in adults. In R. A. Schindler & M. M. Merzenich (Eds.), *Cochlear implants* (pp. 455–460). New York: Raven Press.

Tobey, E. A. (1993). Speech Production. In R. S. Tyler (Ed.), *Cochlear implants: Audiological foundations* (pp. 257–316). San Diego: Singular Publishing.

Tobey, E. A., Geers, A., & Brenner C. (1994). Speech production results: Speech feature acquisition. *Volta Review, 96,* 109–130.

Trammell, J., Farrar, C., Francis, J., Owens, S., Schepard, D., Thies, T., Witlen, R., & Faist, L. (1981). *Test of Auditory Comprehension.* North Hollywood, CA: Foreworks.

Tye-Murray, N. (1992) Conversing with the implanted child. In N. Tye-Murray (Ed.), *Cochlear implants and children: A handbook for parents, teachers and speech and hearing professionals* (pp. 61–78). Washington, DC: A. G. Bell Association for the Deaf.

Tye-Murray, N., & Fryauf-Bertschy, H. (1992). Auditory training. In N. Tye-Murray (Ed.), *Cochlear implants and children: A handbook for parents, teachers and speech and hearing professionals* (pp. 91–114). Washington, DC: A. G. Bell Association for the Deaf.

Tyler, R. S. (1993). *Cochlear implants: Audiological foundations.* San Diego: Singular Publishing.

Tyler, R. S., Berliner, K., Demorest, M., Hirshorn, M., Luxford, W., & Mangham, C. (1986). Clinical objectives and research-design issues for cochlear implants in children. *Seminars in Hearing, 7,* 433–440.

Waltzman, S., Cohen, N., & Shapiro, W. (1994, May). *The effects of cochlear implantation on the young deaf child.* Paper presented at the meeting of the European Symposium on Paediatric Cochlear Implantation, Montpelier, France.

Wilson, B. S. (1993). Signal processing. In R. S. Tyler (Ed.), *Cochlear implants: Audiological foundations* (pp. 35–85). San Diego: Singular Publishing.

Woodcock, K. (1992). Cochlear implants vs. Deaf culture. *Deaf American Monograph, 42,* 151–155.

Zimmerman-Phillips, S., Firszt, J. B., & Kileny, P. R. (1990). Cochlear implant performance in post-meningitis children. *Asha, 32,* 68.

Zimmerman Phillips, S. R., Hieber, S., Zwolan, T. A., Kileny, P. R., Moeggenberg, C., & Telian, S. A. (1994, May). *Changing audiologic criteria in pediatric cochlear implant recipients.* Paper presented at the meeting of the European Symposium on Paediatric Cochlear Implantation, Montpelier, France.

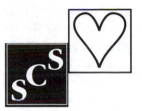

Glossary

Active electrode   The half of the electrode pair that begins stimulation.

A.G. Bell Association for the Deaf   A national organization, located in Washington DC, supporting the use of speech and residual hearing in the oral education of deaf children; members include parents, educators, and hearing-impaired adults and children.

American Sign Language (ASL)   A visual, spatial sign language with a unique grammar and vocabulary.

Auditory learning   Developing speech and language skills through the use of residual hearing in naturalistic exchanges.

Auditory training   Listening exercises often occurring in drill and practice activities.

Bipolar (BP)   The stimulation mode in which the active and indifferent electrodes are beside each other (i.e., #22 = indifferent, #21 = active).

Bipolar plus one (BP+1)   The stimulation mode in which there is one electrode in between the active and indifferent electrodes (i.e., #22 = indifferent, #20 = active).

Bipolar plus two (BP+2)   The stimulation mode in which there are two electrodes in between the active and indifferent electrodes (i.e., #22 = indifferent, #19 = active).

Bipolar plus three (BP+3) The stimulation mode in which there are three electrodes in between the active and indifferent electrodes (i.e., #22 = indifferent, #18 = active).

Chance score The minimum score obtained by guessing at all answers on a standardized test.

Channels The number of separate stimulation sites in the cochlea that can be selectively stimulated. This does not always correspond to the number of electodes.

ChIP The Children's Implant Profile; a protocol for evaluating candidacy for the cochlear implant which reviews factors believed to be related to implant benefit.

Closed set Presentation of all possible choices to the child before giving a test item.

Cochlear Implant Club International An organization for implant users and their families which provides information and support for social, educational, and political purposes.

Comfort level This is the maximum level for a series of pulses that does not produce an uncomfortable loudness sensation for the implant user. These levels are not related to decibels and are commonly called C-Levels in the Nucleus device.

Common ground (CG) This stimulation mode allows for the use of all 22 electrodes. When one electrode is chosen as the active electrode all of the remaining electrodes are connected together and become the indifferent electrode.

Comprehension The highest level of auditory skill development; the ability to respond in a manner which demonstrates that the stimulus was understood.

Compressed analog (CA) This strategy used in the Clarion device incorporates a series of filters which are assigned to different frequencies. The signal is delivered to the appropriate filters depending on the frequency of the incoming sound. Each of these filters is assigned to a pair of electrodes which is stimulated when the signal is sent through the speech processor.

Congenitally deaf Deaf since birth.

Continuous interleaved sampling (CIS) This strategy used in the Clarion device sends the speech signal to the electrodes through a series of very rapid pulses.

Cued speech   A signal system which utilizes hand cues in support of speechreading; cues help to differentiate between and among sounds which look alike on the lips.

Cultural model of deafness   A view of deafness which suggests that deafness is a difference not a deficit and that those who are deaf comprise a subculture with a common language, ASL.

Detection   The ability to hear that a sound is present.

Discourse   Connected sentences which may included a set of directions, a selection from a story or a conversation.

Discrimination   The ability to hear that one sound is the same or different from another.

Duration of deafness   The period of time between the diagnosis of deafness and the age at the time of implantation.

Dynamic range   The number of units between the threshold and comfort levels.

Educational consultant   A teacher of the deaf who provides services to an implant team by acting as the liaison between the medical facility and the local school.

Electrode array   For the Nucleus device, this is made up of 22 electrode bands and 10 retaining rings. The array is designed with the low numbered electrodes (#1) stimulating the high frequency area of the cochlea and the high numbered electrodes (#22) stimulating the low frequency area of the cochlea. For the Clarion device, the electrode array is made up of 16 ball electrodes. These electrodes are placed in pairs and are labelled as being medial or lateral. The array is numbered with the low numbered electrodes (#1) stimulating the low frequency area of the cochlea and the high numbered electrodes stimulating the high frequency area of the cochlea.

Environmental sounds   Nonspeech sounds made by natural and mechanical objects in the environment.

External input of processor   A location on the speech processor in which external devices (telephone, walkman, etc.) can be attached to the speech processor. This area should be kept covered when not in use and cleaned periodically to remove the dust and dirt which accumulates.

Habilitation   Instructional activities designed for the initial teaching of particular skills (e.g., auditory, speech, language).

Identification   The ability to label a stimulus which is heard.

IEP   The Individualized Educational Plan; an annual outline of educational goals and objectives required by law for all children with special needs.

Inclusive education   The education of deaf children supported by special education services in classroom settings with their hearing peers.

Indifferent electrode   The half of the electrode pair that acts as the ground for the electric current.

Interdisciplinary team   A group of professionals from different specialty areas working cooperatively and interdependently for assessment and intervention purposes.

Ling six sounds   Six sounds of English, ah ee, oo, s, sh, m, which are used to determine a child's auditory responsiveness to speech stimuli; they are representative of a range of sounds which occur in conversational speech.

Linguistic environment   The language context in which an auditory target appears.

Listening window   A period of time between the presentation of a stimulus and the child's response to it.

Mainstreaming   The education of deaf children in general school settings with their hearing peers.

Manual communication   A communication methodology which emphasizes a visual representation of language through the use of signs.

Map/mapping   The setting of the Nucleus speech processor according to an individual's measured threshold and comfort levels and subjective responses to sound.

Medical model of deafness   A view of deafness which suggests that it is a pathological condition, that is, the absence of hearing.

Mic input of processor   A location on the Clarion speech processor in which external devices (telephone, walkman, etc.) can be attached. This area should be kept covered when not in use and cleaned periodically to remove the dust and dirt which accumulates.

Monopolar mode   Current which flows between an electrode and an area much further away. The distance between these two areas is much greater than in bipolar mode.

Most comfortable level   This is the maximum level for a series of pulses which does not produce an uncomfortable loudness sensation for the implant user. These levels are not related to decibels and are commonly called M-Levels in the Clarion device.

MPEAK This strategy is the most commonly used in the *MSP* speech processor. It identifies four different parts of the speech signal (known as speech features) and assigns each part to a different electrode.

Multidisciplinary team A group of professionals from different specialty areas contributing individual expertise for assessment and intervention purposes.

NAD The National Association for the Deaf; an organization of deaf adults concerned with social, political, and educational issues of interest to deaf individuals.

NECCI The Network of Educators of Children with Cochlear Implants; an organization of speech and hearing professionals located in New York who have identified themselves as having interest and concern in the education of children with implants.

Open set Presenting a stimulus without previously identifying all possible answers.

Oral communication A communication methodology which emphasizes the use of speech rather than sign for both receptive and expressive exchanges.

Ossification A bony growth within the cochlea, usually as a result of meningitis, which blocks the cochlear turns and prevents full insertion of the electrode array.

Partial insertion The placement of less than the full electrode array in the cochlea. This is generally a result of cochlear ossification or malformation.

Pattern perception The ability to make auditory judgments based on syllable number, word counts in sentences, or stress differences in sentences and connected discourse.

Perilinguistically deafened The loss of hearing during the period of speech and language development (between the ages of 2 and 5 years).

Phoneme An individual speech sound.

Postlinguistically deafened The loss of hearing after the normal development of speech and language (usually age 5 years or older).

Precursor skills Skills that appear developmentally before a particular skill targeted for instruction.

Prelinguistically deafened The loss of hearing before the development of speech and language (may include the congenitally deaf and those deafened before the age of 2 years).

Premarket approval Stage of FDA surveillance which allows a device or drug to be available on a widespread basis.

Processor cord In the Nucleus device, the long cord which connects the microphone to the speech processor. The dot on the cord must match the dot on the microphone for the system to work correctly. In the Clarion device, the long cord which connects the processor to the headpiece.

Productive response A response to a listening task which requires a spoken answer.

Program For the Clarion device, the setting of the speech processor according to an individual's measured threshold and comfort levels and subjective responses to sound.

Program selector A dial on the top of the Clarion speech processor which is numbered from 1–3. This selects the speech processing strategy in use by the patient.

Rehabilitation Instructional activities designed for the reteaching of particular skills (e.g., auditory, speech, language).

Residential school State-supported schools for the deaf with dormitory accommodations; both academic learning and social enculturation of deaf children occurs in this environment.

Segmental speech information Information conveyed by the individual speech sounds of the language.

Sensitivity control The dial on top of the processor which sets the responsiveness of the microphone to the sound source. With a low sensitivity setting the sound source must be very close to the microphone. With a high sensitivity setting, the sound source can be further from the sound source.

Simultaneous communication Speech and sign presented at the same time for both receptive and expressive communication.

SPEAK This strategy is the most recently developed one from the manufacturer of this device and can only be programmed if a child has a *Spectra* speech processor. It identifies the six most prominent peaks of the incoming signal and presents the information to electrodes which correspond to the frequency content of the signal.

Speech perception The ability to understand speech through listening only.

Speechreading Visually scanning the face and especially the lips of the speaker to understand a message.

Speechtracking A speech reading technique which requires the individual to repeat verbtim a paragraph which is being read.

Stimulation mode This determines how much of the electrode array is stimulated each time. When more current is required to obtain T and C levels an increase in the area of stimulation will occur by changing the stimulation mode.

Stimulation units/current level The level of the signal presented through the speech processor. These are the units of current which are delivered through the implant; *decibels are not used* since the signal is an electrical and not acoustical one.

Strategy This determines how the information is sent through the speech processor portion of the implant. The two most common strategies for the Nucleus are called Multipeak *(MPEAK)* and Spectral Peak *(SPEAK)*. The Clarion device uses a Compressed Analog *(CA)* or Continuous Interleaved Sampling *(CIS)*.

Suprasegmental information Information above the level of individual sounds; it includes rhythm, intonation, and stress patterns.

Threshold level The level at which the patient first identifies sound sensation and the lowest level at which the child hears the stimulus every time it is presented. These levels are not related to decibels and are commonly called T-Levels.

Total communication A communication philosophy which suggests that all forms of communication, for example, speech, manual communication, auditory, and speechreading, are available for both receptive and expressive communication.

Transmitter cord The short cord that runs from the microphone to the transmitter coil.

Volume control The dial on the top of the Clarion speech processor which controls the loudness of the sound transmitted to the headset.

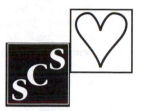

Index

A

A. G. Bell Association, 70, 171
Adolescent user. *See also* Auditory
    learning
  auditory lesson development,
    164–166
  conversation, 164
  coping skills, 163–164
  gains demonstrated, 161–162
  identity development, 162
  networking, 170–171
  nonuse, 162, 170
  postoperative counseling, 168
  self-concept/esteem, 162
  social use, 166
  speech production lesson
    development, 166–167
  speechreading, 163–164, 167–168
  support groups, 170–171
  telecommunication devices for the
    deaf (TTY), 167, 171

  telephone code use, 166–167
  use limited, 169–170
American Sign Language (ASL)
  bilingual/bicultural programs, 96
  Deaf Community, 3
  versus English, 2
  interpreter availability, 6
  residential schools, 6
Americans with Disabilities Act
    (ADA, 1990), 5
Assessment
  auditory perception, 174–176
  device tune-up (external speech
    processor), 74–75
  speech perception, 176–176,
    225–227, 229
  speechreading, 176. *See also* Tests
Audiogram, soundfield, 66
Audiologist, xvi, 56
  educational, 15, 95. *See also*
    Auditory learning
  tune-up (external speech
    processor), 72–78